OSTEOPOROSIS

*How to Make
Your Bones
Last a Lifetime*

**Other Health Titles
from Tribune Publishing**

Aging on Hold

*Cosmetic Surgery:
The Consumer's Complete
Easy Guide from
Before to After*

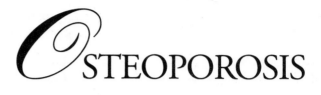STEOPOROSIS

How to Make Your Bones Last a Lifetime

Wanda S. Lyon and
Cynthia E. Sutton

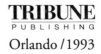

TRIBUNE
PUBLISHING

Orlando / 1993

Copyright © 1993
Wanda S. Lyon and
Cynthia E. Sutton
Illustrations © 1993
Tribune Publishing
75 East Amelia Street
Orlando, Florida 32801

TRIBUNE PUBLISHING
Editorial Director: George C. Biggers III
Managing Editor: Dixie Kasper
Senior Editor: Kathleen M. Kiely
Production Manager: Ken Paskman
Designers: Bill Henderson,
    Eileen M. Schechner, Joy Dickinson

Edited by Kathleen M. Kiely
Text design by Joy Dickinson
Illustrations by Dana Fasano

Thanks to
American Dairy Association
National Dairy Council
Ann Landers, Creators Syndicate
    and *Chicago Tribune*
The National Osteoporosis Foundation
Victor G. Ettinger, M.D., *Recipes for
    Better Bones,* Free from Fat Forever

For information:
Tribune Publishing
P.O. Box 1100
Orlando, Florida 32802

Printed in the United States

FIRST EDITION

Library of Congress Cataloging-in-Publication Data

Lyon, Wanda S.
    Osteoporosis : how to make your bones last a lifetime / by Wanda S. Lyon and
Cynthia E. Sutton. — 1st ed.
        p.   cm.
    Includes bibliographical references and index.
    ISBN 1-56943-005-5
    1. Osteoporosis—Popular works.   I. Sutton, Cynthia E.
II. Title.
RC931.073L94   1993
616.7' 16—dc20   93-28788
                                                  CIP

Contents

To the Reader vii

Acknowledgments viii

1. Osteoporosis: The Preventable Epidemic *1*

2. Caution! Bones at Work *13*

3. Am I at Risk for Osteoporosis? *27*

4. Osteoporosis Screening and Diagnosis *41*

5. Hormones, Menopause and the Great Estrogen Debate *65*

6. Drug Treatments for Osteoporosis *85*

7. Stronger Bodies, Stronger Bones through Physical Activity *107*

8. Fighting Osteoporosis with a Bone-Healthy Diet *153*

9. Great Beginnings: Raising Bone-Healthy Children *195*

10. Injury Prevention: Avoiding Falls and Fractures *207*

*Getting Help: Resources for
Assistance and Information* *215*

Glossary *219*

Select Bibliography *224*

Index *228*

*This book is
dedicated to
our families,
for their patience,
support and love;
and to the countless
men and women
who face the
daily challenge of
living with
osteoporosis.*

To the Reader

*T*his book was written to give you an understanding of one of the most widespread diseases in the world: osteoporosis. Our goal was to provide you with easy-to-read, yet medically accurate, information on up-to-the-minute techniques in osteoporosis prevention, diagnosis and treatment.

A number of medical professionals worked closely with the authors of this book. They spent countless hours poring through the latest information available on osteoporosis. Through this research and interview process we are able to provide you with a diversity of opinion on osteoporosis. This process allows us to present a unique perspective on medical issues: Rather than reading an entire book that reflects one professional opinion, you are receiving information that reflects the thoughts of the top experts in the field. We also talked with another type of expert: the men and women who are living with osteoporosis. They expressed what *you* want and need to know about the disease, and we address your concerns in this book.

The ultimate goal of this book is to provide you with the information you need to make informed decisions about your own health care. We hope you will use the knowledge you gain to become an active partner — along with your doctor — in managing osteoporosis. The information contained in this book is intended to be used as one tool, however, and only in conjunction with advice from your physicians.

Acknowledgments

Our sincere appreciation goes to the health professionals who so graciously provided their time and the in-depth information needed to write this book:

Lenore Hodges, Ph.D., Nutrition, Chief Dietitian, Florida Hospital, Orlando; C. Conrad Johnston, Jr., M.D., professor of Medicine and Director, Division of Endocrinology and Metabolism, Indiana University Medical Center; Wendy Kohrt, Ph.D., Exercise Physiology, Washington University; Robert Lang, M.D., Medical Director of the Osteoporosis Diagnostic and Treatment Centers in New Haven and Bridgeport, Connecticut; Randel K. Miller, M.D., Rheumatology, The Watson Clinic, Lakeland, Florida; B. Lawrence Riggs, M.D., professor of Medical Research at Mayo Medical School and Director of the General Clinical Research Center at the Mayo Clinic in Rochester, Minnesota, and past president of the National Osteoporosis Foundation (1990 through 1992); Sheri Butler, M.A., Exercise Physiology; Walter Earnest, D.P.M.; Penny Glickman, M.D.; Victoria Snyder, R.N.; Jim Treadwell, Sophisticated Imaging Enterprises, Inc., Apopka, Florida.

Our special thanks to these physicians, researchers and other professionals not only for contributing information to this book, but also for their outstanding contributions to women's health. Women will be reaping the rewards of their commitment to the study of osteoporosis for many generations to come.

And, finally, to Kathy Kiely — our editor — and everyone at Tribune Publishing for their commitment to this project.

CHAPTER 1

Osteoporosis: The Preventable Epidemic

*M*illions of women each year are told they have osteoporosis, a disease characterized by bones so weak that they can fracture without warning. These women may feel overwhelmed at first — they are confused and afraid, and often have little understanding of their condition. A recent letter to Ann Landers expressed the concerns and frustrations of many of those whose lives have been affected by osteoporosis:

DEAR ANN LANDERS:
I am a 58-year-old woman and have just been diagnosed with osteoporosis. I went to my doctor because I was having a lot of pain in my back. In addition to the pain, I noticed that I had lost almost 2 inches in my height, and my back, starting at my neck, is beginning to hunch over. It turns out that two of the bones in my spine have not only broken, but they have collapsed and are deteriorating.

My doctor told me I have some of the risk factors for developing osteoporosis, which I didn't know. For instance, I didn't know that since my mother had osteoporosis, I was more likely to get it.

My mother, at age 71, suffered a severe hip fracture which left her permanently disabled. Before this happened, she was active, energetic and young for her age. Today, she is old and frail, uses a walker and can no longer garden, do housework or go out with her friends. She is very dependent on me and my brother, and we worry that the next step will be a nursing home.

I am sure you can understand how upset I am. I have a demanding job and need to be healthy so I can continue to take care of my family responsibilities. What I haven't told you is that I have two daughters who now have a grandmother *and* a mother with this dreadful disease.

My doctor has given me a program that will help me prevent additional fractures. But she also has made it clear that there is no cure for osteoporosis. Once bone mass is lost, it cannot be replaced. On a brighter note, she believes that if I follow my treatment plan, my bone loss will occur at a slower pace.

Ann, I am writing to ask your help. Please tell me where I can get the most reliable information on how to prevent osteoporosis and how I can keep from breaking more bones. I need this information not only for me, but for my children and grandchildren. I want to start early to help them avoid what my mother and I are now going through. When my doctor told me I had osteoporosis, I set out to learn everything I could about the disease, but I have had trouble finding information.

Because this is such a common problem, Ann, there must be millions of people like me who need to be informed. Please help us.

CONCERNED IN NASHVILLE

Concerned in Nashville is right about osteoporosis — there is no cure and it can be difficult to find information and help. But osteoporosis is preventable; with an awareness of her risk factors and a little guidance, *Concerned* might have been able to avoid the fractures she has already suffered. This woman is by no means unique. Osteoporosis is so common in women past the age of menopause that it could have been your mother, aunt or grandmother — or you — writing this letter to Ann Landers.

Osteoporosis is certainly not a new disease; in fact, the term was used to describe bone loss over 50 years ago. Only recently, however, has it been recognized as a condition that can be prevented, and that responds to medical intervention. Though this change has come about slowly, osteoporosis is no longer thought to be an unavoidable result of growing older.

What is Osteoporosis?

Osteoporosis is a condition that exists when the loss of bone over time has caused a drastic weakening of the skeleton. The bones are more than merely a framework over which the rest of the body is draped — they are also the "warehouse" for a number of minerals vital to the everyday functioning of the body. When insufficient levels of these minerals exist in the bloodstream, the body takes action by withdrawing minerals from its skeletal warehouse. If, for any number of reasons, the body is using these minerals without replacing them, the result is a steady decrease in *bone density*. This effect is called *bone loss*, and results in a reduction of the total amount of bone in the body, referred to as *bone mass*.

Researchers have determined that when bone density falls below a certain point, the bones become extremely prone to fracture. This point of impending injury is called the *fracture threshold.* If testing — or, in many cases, a fracture itself — reveals that your bone density has fallen below the fracture threshold, you have *osteoporosis.*

There are two types of osteoporosis. Type I, or primary osteo-porosis, is found in older (postmenopausal) women. This form of osteoporosis is most often manifested by a loss of spongy bone, such as that found in the spine and ribs and in the ends of long bones. Type I is largely the culprit in compression, or crush, fractures of the spine, and in fractures of the wrist. Type II, or secondary osteoporo-sis, is usually seen in patients over the age of 70, or in younger patients who have suffered bone loss as a side effect of another disease or of certain drugs. This form of the disease affects both sexes, but mostly women — in part because they live longer. Type II osteoporosis is manifested by a loss of spongy and hard bone from throughout the skeleton, and is generally at fault in hip fractures.

Many women are shocked when diagnosed with osteoporosis. In

fact, the National Osteoporosis Foundation refers to osteoporosis as "the silent thief" because it usually shows no warning signs. For a number of women, a fracture may be the first indication of the disease. With common detection devices like X-ray, at least 25 percent of a patient's bone mass has to be lost before the disorder can be detected.

An Epidemic of Broken Bones

Medical experts estimate that around 1.5 million broken bones each year are attributable to osteoporosis. Osteoporotic fractures most commonly occur in the bones of the hip, wrist and spine. Bones that

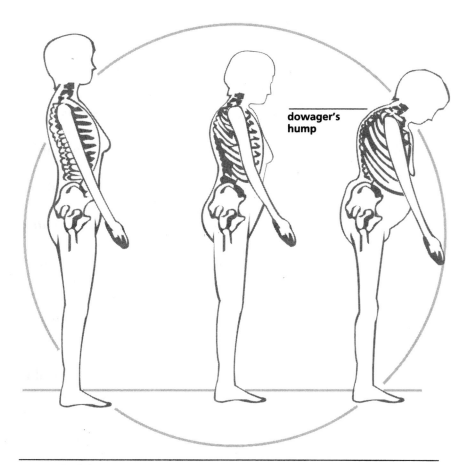

dowager's
hump

How spinal fractures progress

are weakened and brittle from osteoporosis are extremely fragile — crush fractures of the spinal vertebrae are common, and may be brought on by an act as simple as picking up a small grandchild, or stretching to reach a can of peas on the top shelf of the pantry.

Estimates place the number of osteoporotic spinal fractures at approximately half a million a year; statistics tell us that a spinal fracture will be experienced by 40 percent of women by the time they reach 80 years old. Spinal fractures produce the obvious physical signs of osteoporosis: As the vertebrae collapse, the woman (we will use women as examples, since they are the group most affected by osteoporosis) will lose height between the head and

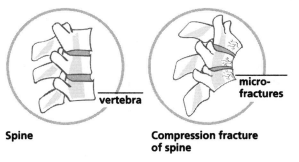

Spine

Compression fracture of spine

pelvis, while the leg bones retain their length. Due to the compacting of the upper body, some women lose several inches of overall height. After several crush fractures, a "dowager's hump" forms between the shoulders due to the outward curvature of the upper spine. As a result, the rib cage may tilt downward, forcing the abdomen to protrude, displacing internal organs and causing extreme discomfort.

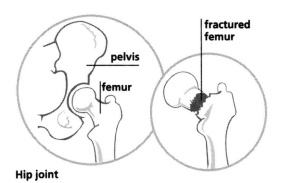

Hip joint

Hip fractures are another serious result of osteoporosis. Fifteen to 20 percent of these injuries ultimately prove to be fatal. While the fracture itself is not generally the direct cause of death, it does set the stage for life-threatening conditions: blood clots, embolisms and pneumonia, for example. Experts estimate that one in three elderly women and one in six elderly men will experience a hip fracture.

A hip fracture generally results from an accident, such as a fall. A person who experiences a hip fracture will probably require an extended stay in the hospital. Many patients require some form of assisted living after release from the hospital, such as a nursing home or a home health aide. In fact, statistics gathered by the Department of Health and Human Services estimate that between 15 and 25 percent of patients who survive a hip fracture will need long-term care.

The Impact of Osteoporosis on Society

Osteoporosis has a huge impact on the women of this country. According to statistics gathered by the National Osteoporosis Foundation, **as many as half of women over the age of 50 will eventually suffer a bone fracture due to osteoporosis**. But this is not just an "old woman's disease" — about one in every three *men* over the age of 75 will be affected by osteoporosis, as well. In fact, approximately one-fifth of osteoporosis patients are men.

As the turn of the millennium approaches, more than 24 million Americans have osteoporosis, and our country is spending an estimated $8 billion to $10 billion each year as a direct result of this disease. The impact of osteoporosis will become even more profound as the oldest of the baby boomers approach menopause, the stage of life when the bone loss that leads to osteoporosis begins to accelerate.

By 2010, more than 60 million American women will be 45 or older. As this huge demographic group ages, osteoporosis statistics can be expected to climb dramatically. In monetary terms, experts estimate that the yearly cost for the care and treatment of osteoporosis patients could reach as much as *$30 billion to $60 billion* in just 30 years. But, as always, baby boomers and the issues that affect them — including osteoporosis — are getting attention.

The Women's Health Initiative

In August 1991, the National Institutes of Health announced the Women's Health Initiative — a 10-year study of the diseases that pose the greatest threat to the lives and physical independence of

American women. These are cardiovascular disease, cancer and osteoporosis. The objective of this study is to identify and test drugs, diet and behavior that may help prevent or forestall these diseases. This enormous effort, which got underway in 1993, has three components:

- Testing new methods of prevention

- Long-term observation to identify new risk factors

- Testing various methods of promoting healthy behavior, through education, community support and use of community resources

The osteoporosis element of the Women's Health Initiative has two main areas of focus: The role of hormone replacement therapy in preventing osteoporosis; and the effect of calcium and vitamin D supplements on prevention.

The clinical trials of the Women's Health Initiative will involve over 55,000 women. Another 100,000 women will be enrolled in a long-term observational study that will try to identify new risk factors for these diseases. These studies will be conducted by selected contractors, such as medical schools and health maintenance organizations (HMOs). Fifteen clinical centers across the country were named in 1993, with another 30 to follow. The study will take about 15 years and more than $600 million to complete. This massive study, along with others already underway, indicates a positive change in the way the research and medical communities — and the United States in general — perceive women's health issues, particularly osteoporosis.

The Good News

More options for the prevention, diagnosis and treatment of osteoporosis exist now than ever before. The development of new methods of detection, coupled with a heightened awareness of this disease on the part of both the public and the medical community, are allowing a much earlier start in arresting the progressive degeneration of bone mass. If you have been diagnosed with osteoporosis, several treatment options are available to help slow your bone loss and possibly save you from further injury, whatever your age or the condition of your skeletal system.

As more and more women take a proactive role in their own health care, many are learning to recognize their risk of osteoporosis and are conveying that concern to their doctors. With proper education and preventive care, you can greatly reduce your chances of developing osteoporosis. If diagnosed, you can take steps to prevent serious injury, call a halt to continuing damage and, if researchers achieve what they are striving for, you may also have the option of taking drugs that will reverse bone loss.

The reason there is good news about osteoporosis today is attributable in great part to men and women like B. Lawrence Riggs, M.D. A professor of Medical Research at Mayo Medical School and Director of the General Clinical Research Center at the Mayo Clinic in Rochester, Minnesota, Dr. Riggs has dedicated over 25 years of his life to the research of osteoporosis, and he served as president of the National Osteoporosis Foundation from 1990 to 1992. It is difficult to find any article on osteoporosis — whether directed to the layperson or the medical professional — without finding some mention of Dr. Riggs and his work. Dr. Riggs was interviewed for this book. When asked what he would like the world to know about osteoporosis, he replied, "I would like people to recognize how common osteoporosis is, the great risk of injury for women with osteoporosis, and that this is a preventable and treatable disease."

Prevention: The Best Medicine

With unanimity, experts agree that the most effective way to deal with osteoporosis is to prevent it — and the first step in prevention is *education*. The National Osteoporosis Foundation, along with other groups and individuals, have devoted themselves to increasing the awareness of osteoporosis. They face the enormous task of educating *both* the medical community *and* the public about the magnitude of the osteoporosis epidemic. Osteoporosis must be brought out of relative obscurity and into the forefront in order to attract the research funding necessary to study it, and to make women aware of their risk.

Dr. Riggs stresses the role of preventive care: "When one woman in two will experience osteoporotic fractures, it is futile to attempt to solve the problem by waiting until fractures occur. The most important aspect of treating osteoporosis is prevention."

Preventing osteoporosis takes a lifetime commitment. In all of life's stages, measures can be taken to protect bone. In childhood, building the greatest possible amount of healthy bone is the goal; later in life, the focus turns to preserving the bone we have.

The Life Stages of Osteoporosis Prevention

A primary goal in preventing osteoporosis is to teach parents how to build strong bones in their children. Parents who are aware of the importance of nutrition and exercise can pass these values on to their children. The residual effect of childhood learning serves as a foundation for more intelligent and bone-healthy choices as young people become adults.

If education is step one in osteoporosis prevention, step two is providing children with the tools they need to build healthy bones. A well-balanced diet rich in calcium and other essential nutrients is crucial. Good nutrition has a partner in building a healthy skeleton: exercise. Experts feel that encouraging children to do what kids do best — run, jump and climb — gives them a "leg up" on developing a strong skeleton. Chapter Nine is devoted to the subject of protecting your children and grandchildren from osteoporosis.

From young adulthood until menopause, the preventive emphasis remains on adequate dietary calcium intake, a program of regular exercise and healthy lifestyle choices, like avoiding cigarettes and caffeine and limiting carbonated beverages and meat. Depending on the level of dietary calcium intake, some adults in this age group are well-advised to begin including calcium supplements in their nutrition plan. See Chapter Eight for in-depth dietary information.

A *perimenopausal* woman (one who has begun to experience some menopausal symptoms) should take a look at where she stands in regard to the risk factors for osteoporosis, and should consider a bone measurement test. Bone loss greatly accelerates during menopause, making it a crucial period in a woman's lifetime effort to maintain healthy bones. "In my practice, I schedule a bone measurement test for all menopausal women, because 50 percent of them will develop osteoporosis," says Robert Lang, M.D., Medical Director of the Osteoporosis Diagnostic and Treatment Centers in New Haven and Bridgeport, Connecticut. A woman identified as having an average or better level of bone density for her age can make an informed decision whether to incorporate estrogen replacement therapy (Chapter Five) into her prevention program. Of course, a woman diagnosed with low bone density would move on to a treatment program that might include estrogen replacement therapy and/or one or more of the drug treatment options discussed in Chapter Six.

As we age, our preventive program must adapt to the normal metabolic changes that occur in our bodies. Older people, including postmenopausal women, must increase their calcium intake, for example, since the body becomes less efficient at storing and processing this vital nutrient. The body's ability to metabolize vitamin D also decreases, making vitamin D supplements a possible component of a prevention program for the elderly. An exercise program may need to be modified to reduce the risk of falling and to limit those types of body movement that can stress fragile bones, such as the twisting actions in tennis and golf.

Everyone, particularly older adults, should take steps to prevent injury in the home, making it free from everyday objects that can contribute to debilitating falls. Simply tripping on a throw rug in the hall can lead to a fall that puts a person in bed for weeks, and this complete lack of physical exercise greatly increases bone loss. "In an environment totally devoid of physical activity, like complete bed rest, the rate of bone loss can accelerate *20- to 50-fold*," cautions Wendy Kohrt, Ph.D., an exercise physiologist at Washington University. "A person can lose the same amount of bone that would normally have been lost in two years in just *two weeks* of complete bed rest."

The rate of bone loss, which accelerates during menopause, usually levels off to about 1 percent per year six to 10 years after menopause. Even though the period of rapid bone loss has already passed, a woman who has not had a bone measurement test during menopause may want to consider one at this point in her life. Once a woman's own rate of bone loss has been determined, patient and doctor can decide whether additional intervention is necessary to prevent the bones from approaching the fracture threshold. The older we get, the more we need help in protecting our skeletons from a significant loss of bone. It is likely at this time in life that the preventive program will evolve into a treatment program, with treatment options called upon to prevent a life-threatening injury and preserve a healthy, active lifestyle.

The Fundamentals of Osteoporosis Prevention

■ Make sure your diet includes 1,000 to 1,500 milligrams of calcium each day. Three 8-ounce glasses of skim milk plus 1 ounce of cheddar cheese provide about 1,100 milligrams of calcium.

■ Consider taking calcium supplements if you are not getting enough dietary calcium every day. One extra-strength Tums antacid provides about 300 milligrams of the type of calcium needed for strong bones. Other types of calcium supplements are available at the vitamin counter. A comparison of calcium supplements can be found in Chapter Eight.

■ Avoid eating large amounts of meat, smoking cigarettes and drinking excessive caffeinated or alcoholic beverages, especially if you have a low calcium intake. Don't eat foods high in insoluble fiber along with those foods or beverages that you depend on to provide your dietary calcium.

■ Exercise, exercise, exercise. Weight-bearing exercises such as walking help maintain bone. Aim for 30 to 60 minutes per day, three to five times per week. Try to mix in some other types of exercise for maximum bone benefit. Increasing the intensity of weight-bearing exercises will reap aerobic benefit and maintains cardiovascular health. (See Chapter Seven for more information on the importance of exercise.)

■ Relax in the sunshine for 15 minutes every day to get your recommended 400 I.U. (international units) of vitamin D. Avoid supplements that exceed 400 I.U. per day, because a significant excess of vitamin D may be toxic and can actually cause bone *loss*.

■ Consider a bone measurement test around the age of menopause, and follow up as advised by your doctor. Make certain that you understand all aspects of estrogen replacement therapy so that you can make an informed decision.

■ Check your home for objects and situations that increase your risk of falling, such as dark halls and stairways and slippery throw rugs. (Chapter Ten includes important safety tips.)

In a 1987 interview, Dr. Riggs expressed optimism that osteoporosis would be brought under control within 10 years. As we close in on that 10-year mark, have the years dimmed his hopes that this can be accomplished? "I think we have made huge progress, and it is still realistic to expect that [osteoporosis will be brought under control]," he says. "But by under control I don't mean eliminated like smallpox, but rather [controlled] like high blood pressure, where you can diagnose it early, you can put people on treatment and you can prevent complications of the disease. I see that happening within five more years."

A *sound mind in a sound body, is a short but full description of a happy state in the world.*

JOHN LOCKE,
Some Thoughts Concerning Education (1693)

Locke's poetic phrasing embraces a universal thought: The prospect of living out our years with a healthy mind *and* a healthy body is a goal we would all like to achieve. Our bones work hard throughout our lives. In all of life's stages, we can take positive steps that will enable our skeletal system to continue its work, giving us the opportunity to enjoy a sound mind and a sound body for many, many years.

CHAPTER 2

Caution!
Bones at Work

*O*ur bones *are* at work — all day, every day, for our entire lives. They perform tasks critical to the normal functioning of our bodies, such as the manufacture of blood and storage of nutrients, and the bones themselves are continually being taken apart and rebuilt in a process appropriately called *remodeling*.

Let's take a moment for a basic anatomy lesson: The skeletal system is made up of 206 separate bones. These bones form the foundation of the body, providing us with our most fundamental physical shape (tall, short, petite, large-boned) and protecting our vital organs, as in the manner the skull protects the brain. Our skeleton is held together at the joints by bands of tissue called *ligaments*. We are able to move our limbs and bodies because of the *muscles* attached to our bones by strong cord-like fibrous tissues called *tendons*.

All bones are encased in a thin, tough, protective membrane of tissue called the *periosteum*, except at the joints where there is a layer of *cartilage*. A fibrous, flexible tissue, cartilage plays an important part in skeletal processes. An infant's skeleton is made up primarily of cartilage, which gradually hardens as crystals of *calcium phosphate* become embedded in it. Cartilage is an integral part of the mechanism by which bones grow in length, called *longitudinal growth*. Longitudinal growth occurs at the ends of bones, where there are thin disks of cartilage called *epiphyseal growth plates*. During periods of growth in childhood and adolescence, cartilage grows over existing hard bone, then the cartilage itself gradually hardens from the deposits of calcium phosphate, becoming bone. A new layer of cartilage forms on this newly formed bone, which in turn hardens, and so on. Adult height is reached when the growth plates stop functioning.

Beneath the protective sheath of the periosteum lies the outer layer of bone, called compact or *cortical* bone. This hard, dense shell of bone is the primary component in such long bones as the femur of the thigh. *Trabecular* bone, which has a cancellous, or spongy, texture, makes up the inner layer of bone tissue. It is softer and more porous than cortical bone, and makes up a large part of the vertebrae and ribs.

Not only do our bones protect our vital organs, support our bodies and provide us with mobility, they also store the body's supply of calcium. In fact, 99 percent of the body's supply of calcium is stored in the skeleton, with the majority of this calcium reservoir residing in the trabecular tissues. As part of the bone remodeling process, the calcium stored in bones is released into the bloodstream, where it is used throughout the body for such critical

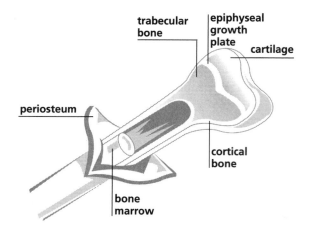

functions as the proper clotting of blood, maintenance of the heartbeat, and normal functioning of muscles and nerves.

Bone marrow is found in the hollow cavities deep in the interior of the bones. It is composed of blood vessels and a network of tissue fibers containing fat and the cells that produce blood. Both red and white blood cells are manufactured in bone marrow and are released into the bloodstream when fully developed. In times of crisis, bone marrow will speed up the manufacture of the type of blood cells needed: If an infection threatens the body, marrow steps up production, turning out more white blood cells. In cases of anemia or hemorrhage, bone marrow produces more red blood cells.

Two types of marrow are found in our bones: *Red marrow* is involved in the production of the blood cells; *yellow marrow* is mostly fat tissue. Red marrow is most abundant in the early years of our lives, with the fatty yellow marrow gradually taking over as we age and our blood-production needs decrease. A small supply of red marrow will remain at selected sites in the skeleton throughout our lives, however, and our bodies will convert yellow marrow to red if a time of crisis increases the need for blood cell production.

All the bones in the skeleton are made up of nerves, blood vessels, marrow, and a combination of both cortical and trabecular bone tissue. However, the proportion of each type of bone tissue varies throughout the skeletal system. The vertebrae in the spine, for example, consist primarily of the softer, sponge-like trabecular bone surrounded by a thin layer of the harder, denser cortical bone. In contrast, many of the long bones in the arms and legs are made up almost entirely of hard cortical bone, with much smaller amounts of the more porous trabecular tissue within. The femur (thigh bone), for example, is nearly three-quarters cortical bone. The total amount of both types of bone in the entire skeleton is called *bone mass.* The level of bone mass is critical to the health and strength of the skeleton. Changes in *bone density,* brought on by various factors, can cause increases and decreases in bone mass throughout life.

Bone Remodeling: The Cycle of Skeletal Renewal

Bone is continuously formed, broken down and formed again by the *bone remodeling process.* Bone remodeling is at work throughout your skeletal system right now — on a microscopic level, minute areas of old bone are being removed and new bone is being produced. This remodeling cycle keeps bones strong and healthy, and it also releases calcium stored in the bones for use throughout the body. There are several key components in bone remodeling, each reliant on the others to perform its task. These components work together in a process to manufacture and maintain bone tissue.

The actual breaking down and rebuilding of bone tissue is performed by two specialized groups of cells. The first group, which handles the destruction of existing bone, are called *osteoclasts.* Osteoclasts work by dissolving tiny areas of existing bone tissue, freeing the calcium to be reabsorbed, or *resorbed,* into the blood stream. The entire bone removal process is referred to as *bone resorption.*

It can take as long as three or four months for the remodeling process to complete its cycle, but this resorption phase of bone remodeling clips along at a relatively rapid pace. Osteoclasts usually complete their job in as little as a week to 10 days, leaving behind minute cavities in the bone. The osteoclasts then signal the bone-building cells to begin their job.

I n adults, up to one-third of the body's bone is replaced each year by the bone remodeling process. That means that as much as 30 percent of your skeleton is less than one year old!

The bone-building cells that fill the tiny craters created by the resorption process are called *osteoblasts.* Osteoblasts deposit a matrix made up primarily of a protein called *collagen.* As a matter of fact, the collagen matrix deposited by the osteoblasts has the same basic composition as the collagen that is part of your skin tissues.

Within two weeks the soft collagen matrix will begin to go through a hardening or *mineralization* phase. During this phase of the remodeling process, *calcium* and *phosphorus* from the bloodstream become embedded in the collagen matrix in the form of calcium phosphate crystals. This mineralization phase of bone remodeling makes up a large proportion — about 65 percent — of the total bone remodeling process.

This deposit of calcium phosphate during the mineralization phase contributes to the *density* of the bones. *Bone density* refers to the volume of calcium within the bone tissue. As we age, the loss of calcium results in bones that are less dense and more porous. Measuring the total calcium content of the bones indicates *bone mineral content* (BMC).

The Effect of Hormones on Bone

The delicately balanced process of bone remodeling is regulated to a large extent by various hormones. Some of these hormones act as "traffic cops," controlling the activity of the bone-destroying and bone-building cells, while other hormones act directly on the bone tissue itself. The *growth hormone* produced by the pituitary gland helps stimulate the remodeling cycle; *calcitonin,* a thyroid hormone, helps repress the bone-destroying osteoclasts. *Parathyroid hormone* stimulates osteoclast activity, helps convert vitamin D to an active form that increases dietary calcium absorption, and helps the kidneys metabolize calcium. Sex hormones, such as *estrogen* and *progesterone*, act as bone protectors in a number of ways, one of which is by preventing *adrenal hormones* from destroying bone.

Even the bone-friendly hormones aren't always so amiable, however. Too much or too little of several of these hormones can have a significant negative effect on bone mass. For example, excess parathyroid or thyroid hormones can result in bone loss due to overzealous osteoclast (bone-destroying) activity.

Sex hormones like estrogen, progesterone and, in males,

androgens spur rapid growth in adolescence. During those years, a variety of hormones stimulate the bone-building cells to form far greater amounts of new bone at an accelerated pace, much faster than the bone-destroying cells can break them down. The reverse is also true: In the years during menopause, declining levels of estrogen and progesterone can result in the loss of valuable bone mass. The effect of hormones on the remodeling process has become the focus of much research being done on the prevention and treatment of osteoporosis and other bone disorders.

The bone remodeling cycle proceeds at its own pace for each individual, resulting over time in the replacement of old bone with new, called *bone turnover.* Some people have a high rate of bone turnover, while in others the process moves more slowly. Even different parts of the skeleton undergo various rates of remodeling. However, the crucially important factor in building and maintaining bone mass is the *ratio* of the amount of bone resorption to the amount of bone formation: **When more bone is being built than destroyed, bone mass and density can increase; when the amount of bone being broken down is *greater* than the amount being formed, bone mass is lost.**

Left to its own devices, the bone remodeling balance will tilt throughout our lives for a variety of reasons, with the most fundamental reason being the changes that come with age.

Childhood and Adolescence: The Growing Years

A great deal of activity goes on in the skeletal system during the pre-adult phase of our lives. Bone-building cells are working rapidly to replace cartilage with bone, forming much more new bone than the bone-destroying cells can keep pace with. Most of this growth is longitudinal, taking place at the bone growth plates.

The most rapid period of growth in childhood takes place in the first two years of a child's life. In the first year, a typical infant grows about *eight inches* — more than a third of its birth length. Year two is nearly as impressive, with typical growth of about five inches. And consider the amount the fetus has grown while still in the mother's womb: During 40 to 42 weeks of pregnancy, the child has developed a skeletal system that results in a birth height between 18 and 26 inches. Therefore, in the period of time since conception, a two-year-old child has grown between 31 and 39 inches!

The teenage years spur a second period of accelerated bone growth. At the onset of puberty, a young person's hormones seem to "go crazy." This sudden infusion of sex hormones, which has brought terror to parents of teenagers throughout time, serves a critical function for the skeletal system: It stimulates bone growth. In natural symmetry, the body's ability to absorb and metabolize the nutrients necessary for bone building also peaks at this age. During this phase of "all systems go," the bone remodeling process and all the contributing systems of the body are functioning at optimum capacity.

Reaching the Peak

At a certain point in life, bones reach their maximum density and strength. This state of maximum density is called *peak bone mass*. The two different types of bone tissue, cortical and trabecular, reach their peaks separately. Trabecular bone, as the storehouse of the body's calcium supply, is subjected to more intense metabolic activity. Perhaps as a result, it reaches its peak relatively early in life. Cortical bone, on the other hand, continues to build mass after trabecular bone has reached its peak.

Until fairly recently, experts believed that peak bone mass was achieved between the ages of 25 and 40. Developments in the techniques for measuring bone mass have changed that opinion, however. B. Lawrence Riggs, M.D., professor of Medical Research at Mayo Medical School and director of the General Clinical Research Center at the Mayo Clinic in Rochester, Minnesota, explains: "New densitometry [measurement of bone density] data has changed estimates on the age at which we reach peak bone mass. The old data, which indicated that 30 to 35 was the age of peak bone mass, was based on cortical width measurements and hand X-rays made 30 years ago. Today, we feel that you reach the peak of [trabecular] bone, which is the more metabolically active bone, around 15 or 20

The Four Phases of Bone Mass

■ **Skeletal Growth: Conception to 18 Years Old**
The amount of new bone formed exceeds the amount of old bone destroyed, resulting in longitudinal growth.

■ **Peak Bone Mass: 15 to 30 Years Old**
The bone remodeling process is in near perfect balance. Bone goes through a consolidation phase, in which maximum lifetime bone density and strength are achieved.

■ **Age-Related Bone Loss: 35 to 40 Years and Older**
The body becomes less efficient at absorbing and metabolizing calcium and vitamin D, and natural changes occur in the remodeling process that result in loss of bone mass.

■ **The Menopause Effect: Onset of Menopause**
The decline in the level of estrogen in the system contributes to a phase of accelerated bone loss that peaks in the first four to eight years after the onset of menopause. Rate of bone loss slowly stabilizes and resumes the slower rate of bone loss related to aging.

years of age, then the epiphyses [growth plates] close and you stop growing. Although there is some filling out of cortical bone for another 10 years or so, about 70 percent of our bone mass is accumulated in the adolescent years."

The level of density attained at peak bone mass is the key to continued skeletal health. The two most important indicators of whether an individual will suffer from osteoporosis are the amount of bone tissue accumulated at the time of peak bone mass, and the rate at which bone mass is lost after this peak period. **To achieve maximum benefit, adults must begin to control loss of bone mass between the ages of 25 and 40.** We get no second chances when it comes to maintaining peak bone mass. When it's gone, it's gone.

The Adult Years

As we enter our twenties, the phase of longitudinal bone growth that took place in the first and second decades of life comes to an end, and the body enters into a brief period of bone consolidation, in which bone density increases. When we are in our twenties and thirties, the remodeling process is in near-perfect harmony. The ratio of bone resorption to bone formation is balanced — the amount of old bone broken down by the osteoclasts is in parity with the amount of new bone built by the osteoblasts.

Trabecular bone, the primary component of the spine, begins to lose mass between the ages of 25 and 30.

Beginning at about age 40, bone resorption slowly begins to overtake bone formation in the total remodeling process, in both men and women. The result is a gradual but constant loss of bone mass that will continue throughout the remainder of one's life. Though this loss of bone is experienced by everyone, the rate of loss differs in individuals and between the sexes. The decline in bone mass is attributed to several factors, among them decreased calcium absorption, decline in the efficiency of the bone-building phase of the remodeling process and, in some cases, a deficiency of vitamin D. At the root of all these contributing factors: *age.*

After age 35 to 40, the age-related loss of bone density begins, and will be accelerated during menopause. Men begin losing bone mass about 10 years later than women, at a fairly constant rate (about 1 percent per year) throughout the remainder of their lives.

In addition to the obvious disadvantage of losing bone mass through the natural course of aging, the rate of bone turnover also slows as we get older. That means the bones themselves get *older*, because the remodeling process does not replace old bone with new bone as rapidly as it did when we were younger. Older bones may be more likely to suffer stress fractures and tiny microcracks, further weakening the skeletal structure as a whole.

The illustrations below demonstrate the degenerative changes in bone tissue that can result in osteoporosis. The holes or spaces in the healthy bone on the left are the normal porous nature of trabecular bone. The bone on the right shows a marked decrease in density, because the tissue has lost significant amounts of the calcium phosphate that had been deposited in it. This *loss of mineralization* is what weakens bones and leads to osteoporosis.

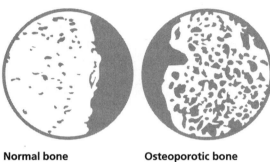

Normal bone   **Osteoporotic bone**

The erosion of bone mass is an unwanted but natural result of growing older, and can result in the development of osteoporosis in men and women as aging continues. Unfortunately for women, the added effects of menopause and the resulting changes in the female body fan the flames of bone loss.

The Effects of Menopause on Bone

When a woman reaches her late forties or early fifties, she can antici-pate the beginning of *menopause,* sometimes called the "change of life." The medical term for the symptoms of menopause is *climac-teric.* During menopause, a woman's body undergoes a series of chemical alterations, the most notable of which are declining levels of estrogen and progesterone in her system. Hot flashes, night sweats, irregular menstrual periods, fatigue, weight gain and depres-sion can be experienced by a woman during menopause; she must also be aware of the very real threat to her skeletal system caused by accelerated bone loss.

Our Friend FAT

*Y*es, good old fat — most of us seem to have it in unwanted abundance. But fat does have at least one redeeming feature: It helps the body produce estrogen.

Following menopause, the amount of estrogen manufactured by the ovaries dwindles to nearly nothing. However, the ovaries, along with the adrenal glands, do continue to produce the male sex hormones, androgens. Our friend fat takes the androgens produced by the ovaries and adrenal glands and converts it into bone-preserving estrogen.

Throughout a woman's life, from the time she starts menstruating until menopause, her ovaries produce estrogen. Estrogen is a "bone friendly" hormone, meaning that it helps the body maintain bone mass. Many studies have been done on the effects of estrogen on the bone remodeling process, but researchers have just recently started to uncover the mysteries of how the hormone works to protect bone mass, and some of the exact mechanisms are still unclear.

When the ovaries slow their production of estrogen, either naturally or in the case of *surgical menopause* (a *hysterectomy* with *oophorectomy*, removal of the ovaries along with the uterus) the major source of a much-needed bone protector is gone. While some estrogen will continue to be produced in a conversion process that takes place in fat tissue, the supply of estrogen available to ward off bone loss is drastically diminished.

Researchers believe that one of the crucial ways estrogen benefits bone is that it helps keep the osteoclasts from becoming over-industrious and breaking down more bone than the osteoblasts can rebuild. Estrogen and progesterone also repress the negative effect of adrenal and parathyroid hormones, which can actually destroy bone as well as signaling the body to speed up the resorption process. The decline in estrogen level experienced with menopause and ovary removal surgery nearly eliminates these benefits, and reduces the body's ability to absorb and use calcium and vitamin D, two of the most crucial bone building blocks.

Chapter One introduced the two types of osteoporosis: Type I occurs in postmenopausal women; Type II is seen in both sexes and is the result of aging. Unfortunately, women are not subject to just one type at a time — the loss of bone that brings on Type I osteoporosis actually occurs *simultaneously* with the Type II effects of aging on bone. Therefore, a woman experiencing menopause undergoes a lengthy period of significantly accelerated bone loss; a period of "double jeopardy."

A fter attaining peak bone mass in the years following adolescence, a woman loses about 35 percent of her cortical bone and about 50 percent of her trabecular bone during her lifetime.

The greatest loss of bone mass occurs in the first four to eight years after the onset of menopause, then the rate of loss begins to decline until it levels off to the normal age-related loss rate. Some women, however, can experience increased bone loss due to declining levels of estrogen for as long as *20 years*. Experts believe that women lose 10 percent of cortical bone mass and another 25 percent of trabecular bone mass as a result of estrogen deficiency resulting from menopause. In their lifetime, women will lose a total of about 35 percent of their peak cortical bone mass and 50 percent of their peak trabecular bone mass. Men, however, will lose about 25 percent of cortical bone mass and 33 percent of trabecular bone mass in their lifetime, approximately two-thirds the amount of loss in peak bone mass experienced by women.

A key health decision a woman may have to make in her lifetime is whether to undergo *estrogen replacement therapy (ERT)*. ERT has engendered heated debate within the medical community, among researchers and among women themselves. In a nutshell, ERT is acknowledged to be a strong preventive treatment for osteoporosis. The downside, however, is that some research indicates an increased risk of certain types of cancer among patients undergoing estrogen replacement therapy. More in-depth information on estrogen and its effect on bone mass is found in Chapter Five.

The Senior Years

The changes and choices that menopause brings to a woman's life greatly affect the health of her bones. In addition, a number of other changes that take place in the bodies of aging women and men alike can spell trouble for the bones.

Aging impairs the body's ability to absorb and metabolize calcium and vitamin D from the diet. Calcium performs key functions in the body in addition to building bone: It regulates the heartbeat, provides normal transmission of nerve impulses, aids in muscle contraction and facilitates normal clotting of the blood. When the calcium in the diet is insufficient to maintain these vital functions, or if the calcium is poorly absorbed, the body will begin to draw on the calcium reservoir stored in the bones. Thus the body steps up bone resorption to put needed calcium into the bloodstream. Result: loss of bone mass.

As we get older, all the systems of the body have slower repair capabilities. Illnesses like a cold or the flu can take longer to get over. The prolonged period of bed rest that may be necessary at this age to recuperate from an illness can have an adverse effect on the bones: Even a few days of complete inactivity can cause a significant decline in bone mass. In addition, an individual who has spent a few days restricted to bed may feel weak and dizzy upon becoming mobile again, causing serious risk for a bone-injuring fall. A fall would likely result in more bed rest, and a vicious cycle begins.

Age and gender are the two aspects of our lives that have the greatest impact on whether we develop osteoporosis. While the march of time is inevitable, and our gender and family tree are virtually cast in stone, there are ways to slow the degenerative effect on our bones from accumulated birthdays and inherited genes. Likewise, a number of lifestyle factors increase or decrease the odds of contracting this disease — and changes we can make in our daily lives may swing the odds of developing osteoporosis in our favor.

One of the basic prerequisites to winning this war is to recognize the enemy. In Chapter Three, you will learn to recognize those aspects of lifestyle and heredity that increase your personal level of risk for osteoporosis. Once you have identified the enemy, you can effectively plan the strategy for your war on osteoporosis.

CHAPTER 3

Am I at Risk for Osteoporosis?

A trusted friend stops by to visit. Gently, she takes your hand and looks into your eyes. She informs you that she has received information of a threat to your health and well-being. This threat could cause you injury and change the way that you live, but it *can* be avoided if you take proper action now. Would you want your friend to tell you what that threat is, and how you can prevent it?

The information in the following pages is going to help you determine whether there is a threat to your health and well-being lurking in the future. Osteoporosis threatens the health and independence of millions of people each year, but *it is preventable.* **The first step in avoiding osteoporosis is to determine your level of risk for the disease.**

While a number of factors contribute to the development of osteoporosis, the single most predominant factor is age. Loss of bone mass is a natural result of aging, beginning for women at about age 30. Without preventive action, from that point until menopause a woman will lose bone mass at a rate of about .5 to 1 percent per year. During the first six to eight years of menopause that rate will increase to a range of 2 to 10 percent per year. In her lifetime, a woman will lose about 50 percent of the type of bone that makes up much of her spine, if steps are not taken to intervene in the natural rate of loss. Experts estimate that over 40 percent of women and over 17 percent of men who survive to age 90 will experience a hip fracture, and a majority (up to 90 percent!) of women will be clinically osteoporotic by age 75.

Frightening numbers, aren't they? But there *is* reason for optimism, because osteoporosis does not have to be a part of your life. You can identify those aspects of your lifestyle and certain inherited characteristics that put you at risk for developing osteoporosis, and take action to work against them. While you may not be able to stop the aging process, you can certainly take preventive steps that will keep you from becoming one of the grim statistics.

While most of the factors that cause osteoporosis develop as we get older, bone fractures attributed to the effects of osteoporosis have been reported in premenopausal women and even in children. Osteoporosis among these groups, however, is almost always due to rare circumstances such as some form of bone disease, like *osteitis fibrosa,* which is caused by an overactive parathyroid gland. In this condition, a hormone stimulates the bone-destroying cells to break down more bone tissue than can be formed by the bone-building cells, resulting in severe loss of bone mass. Children can suffer a softening of the bones, familiarly called *rickets,* which results in deformities such as "bow legs." In adults this condition is called *osteomalacia,* and is essentially a breakdown in the mineralization process that hardens bone.

Several other factors can contribute to osteoporosis in premenopausal women and other young people:

■ A chronically excessive physical exercise program that has brought on *amenorrhea,* or the cessation of menstruation. This condition is most often seen in female athletes and dancers, and results in loss of the protective effects of estrogen.

■ A severe eating disorder such as *bulimia* or *anorexia nervosa,* in which the patient has become extremely and chronically malnourished.

■ Long-term treatment with certain prescription drugs such as anti-convulsants, corticosteroids and thyroid medication.

■ Faddish vegetarian diets (high fiber, little or no calcium intake) or other diets extremely lacking in nutrients essential to building and maintaining bone mass.

While osteoporosis is much more of a threat to older people than to the young, it is in their early years that many osteoporosis patients laid the groundwork for severe bone loss later in life. In fact, the precursor of osteoporosis is a condition called *osteopenia,* which can be found in people of any age. Osteopenia is simply abnormally low bone mass that has not yet weakened the bone to the *fracture threshold,* at which bones are so lacking in density that spontaneous fractures can occur.

We have a limited number of years in which to build our bone mass to its peak. Once we have reached the age of 35 to 40, the remainder of our lives will be spent attempting to maintain as much of our bone as possible, and to slow the natural degeneration that will inevitably occur if preventive measures are not taken.

The Risks of Osteoporosis

According to statistics gathered by the National Osteoporosis Foundation:

■ A woman's risk of suffering a hip fracture is equal to the combined risks of her developing breast, uterine and ovarian cancer.

■ Nearly 70,000 Americans each year will require the help of a continued-care facility (such as a nursing home) due to the effects of a hip fracture.

Osteoporosis usually results from a combination of several risk factors. Some of these are *controllable* behavioral or environmental factors; things *you* can change. Other factors are *unavoidable;* either inherited in the genes passed down to you from your parents, or the result of a physical disorder.

Unavoidable Risk Factors

Aging is the universal factor that leads to osteoporosis. A number of other unavoidable factors can compound the effects of aging, greatly predisposing an individual to developing osteoporosis. The first step in forming your battle plan against this disease is to know the extent of the threat to you. The unavoidable factors are:

GENDER   If you are female, you are a prime candidate for osteoporosis simply by virtue of your sex. Women have about 25 percent less bone mass at its peak than their male counterparts. Add to that the naturally accelerated rate of bone loss following menopause (due to the loss of valuable bone-saving hormones) and it is not difficult to figure out why women are, overall, about eight times more likely to be affected by osteoporosis than men. In addition, men generally have higher levels of the hormones that help maintain bone density. The National Osteoporosis Foundation cites studies indicating that up to half of American women over age 45 will be affected by osteoporosis. Finally, since women have a longer life expectancy than men, they are more likely to develop age-related osteoporosis.

RACE   People who have inherited fair skin are much more likely to become osteoporotic than those with a darker complexion. Researchers have found that light-skinned women whose ancestors originated from northern Europe, the United Kingdom, Japan, China and other regions of the Far East are at more risk than women who are of Hispanic, African and Mediterranean ancestry. Racially, Caucasians and Asians are at the highest risk. Persons with a black African heritage have heavier bone density, amounting to about 10 to 15 percent higher bone mass than fairer-skinned people.

Consequently, black women over the age of 60 have about one-half the incidence of hip fractures as white women of the same age.

BODY SIZE   Small-boned women are at greater risk for developing osteoporosis due to a relatively low peak bone mass. And lower body weight means less physical stress on your bones in carrying you around — the type of stress that makes your bones more dense. Petite women have less bone going into the years in which they will begin to lose bone density.

By the same principle, thin individuals or women with a low percentage of body fat also face a higher risk. Small-boned and thin are *not* the same thing: A woman may be large-framed and have a low percentage of body fat. While some women may argue otherwise, there is a positive aspect to having a higher percentage of body fat: Fat helps produce estrogen, and estrogen has been proven to slow bone loss. Therefore, lean women are more prone to osteoporosis due to a lower estrogen level. Keep in mind, however, that a higher percentage of body fat may increase the risk for other conditions, such as heart disease and certain kinds of cancer.

FAMILY HISTORY   If someone in your family tree has had osteoporosis or another bone disease, you are much more likely to be affected by the same condition. If older women in your family have suffered fractures attributable to osteoporosis, be especially alert to your increased risk. Such a history also puts your daughters at higher risk.

MENOPAUSE   Postmenopausal women are extremely prone to osteoporosis: As many as *half* of the women who experience natural menopause will develop the disorder. *Early menopause*, either natural or surgical (caused by removal of the ovaries), has been cited by the National Osteoporosis Foundation as one of the strongest predictors of osteoporosis. (An early menopause is one that begins before age 45.)

Why is menopause such a turning point? Because when the ovaries stop producing the hormones estrogen and progesterone, the bones lose a valuable ally in fighting bone loss. Estrogen helps protect bone from numerous "bone-stealers," even other hormones within the body.

DISEASE   Individuals who suffer from certain diseases that affect bone mass face an increased risk of osteoporosis. Most of these diseases act on the body's ability to process, absorb and store the nutrients essential for maintaining healthy bone tissue. In addition, the medications prescribed in the treatment of some of these diseases may interfere with the body's ability to achieve a normal peak bone mass. Among these conditions are:

Thyroid disease   An overactive thyroid gland stimulates the osteoclasts, or bone-destroying cells, in the bone remodeling process. These cells begin to do their job too aggressively, breaking down more bone than can be rebuilt in the normal process. As a result, the patient loses bone mass and eventually becomes osteoporotic.

Stomach, intestinal or bowel disorders   Many digestive tract conditions interfere with the body's ability to absorb and metabolize calcium and other nutrients essential for healthy bone.

Liver or kidney disease   Both liver and kidney disease can prevent the body from absorbing and processing adequate calcium to build and maintain healthy bone tissue. In addition, kidney disease can lead to unhealthy levels of acids and phosphate in the blood, both of which are harmful to bones.

Parathyroid disease   Hormones secreted by the tiny parathyroid glands help regulate the amount of bone broken down to provide calcium to the rest of the body. These hormones also tell the kidneys when more calcium is needed in the bloodstream, and they help activate vitamin D so that calcium is better absorbed and processed for bone building. Too much *or* too little of the parathyroid hormones are harmful to bone.

The Risk for Osteoporosis: What Factors Are Controllable?

Unavoidable factors that increase the risk for osteoporosis

Aging	White or Asian ancestry
Female gender	Family history of osteoporosis
Menopause	Small-boned or petite frame
Certain diseases	Certain medications

Controllable factors that can contribute to osteoporosis

Caffeine	Alcohol
Smoking	Carbonated beverages
Not enough calcium	Inadequate exercise
Diet heavy in salt, animal protein or fiber	Excessive exercise resulting in cessation of menstruation

MEDICATIONS   Certain drugs are known to contribute to loss of bone mass. Patients taking these medications may wish to have a conversation with their doctors about the relationship between these drugs and osteoporosis. Some of the more common medications that have an adverse effect on bone mass are:

Anticonvulsants   Some of these drugs affect the body's ability to absorb and process vitamin D in the liver. They lead to vitamin D deficiency, reducing the amount of calcium made available and resulting in loss of bone mass.

Thyroid medication   Research indicates that even small overdoses of thyroid hormones can increase risk of osteoporosis.

Corticosteroids   Millions of patients are treated with these drugs for asthma and rheumatoid arthritis. These medications decrease the formation of new bone and also have a negative effect on calcium absorption. Extended use of corticosteroids such as cortisone, prednisolone, hydrocortisone and dexamethasone can result in osteoporosis.

Controllable Risk Factors

Though you may have several of the unavoidable risk factors for osteoporosis, thoughtful management of your behavior and your environment — that is, your overall lifestyle — can tip the balance against your developing the disease. How you live your life will make a considerable difference in the severity of bone loss and the age at which osteoporosis develops, if at all. **Your behavior and environment are factors that you can control.**

The lifestyle choices listed here have been strongly implicated as contributing to the development of osteoporosis. Study after study has revealed a much higher incidence of osteoporosis in people whose lives include these factors:

ALCOHOL Excessive consumption of alcohol (three or more drinks per day) has been firmly linked to the development of osteoporosis. Numerous studies indicate that even *small* amounts of alcohol interfere with the normal processing and absorption of both calcium and Vitamin D, and diminish the body's ability to build and maintain bone mass. **Alcohol is the number one factor in the development of osteoporosis in men.** Individuals who are at heightened risk for osteoporosis due to other factors should be especially vigilant in controlling their consumption of alcoholic beverages.

In addition to the direct negative effect that alcohol has on the formation of healthy bone tissue, drinking too much alcohol can also contribute to osteoporosis in other, more subtle ways: People who drink heavily are more apt to have poor nutritional habits and to avoid physical exercise.

CAFFEINE   Even though you may enjoy that morning cup of coffee and the "jump start" it gives you in taking on the challenges of the day, your bones will thank you if you switch to a decaffeinated brand. In a joint study on thousands of elderly patients, researchers at several Northeastern universities found that drinking substantial amounts of caffeinated beverages (equal to the caffeine in three-and-one-half cups of coffee or seven cups of tea per day) nearly *doubles* the risk of developing osteoporosis. The study helped researchers confirm the belief that caffeine interferes with the normal bone remodeling process and contributes to the loss of calcium through the urine.

While the effects on bone mass attributable to caffeine are still being studied, the indications are clear: Cutting back or eliminating caffeine from your diet reduces your risk of osteoporosis.

SMOKING   It seems there is yet another excellent reason for abstaining from this habit. In addition to the risks of heart disease, lung disease and several kinds of cancer, it is now known that smokers face an increased risk of developing osteoporosis.

Study after study has shown a greater incidence of osteoporosis in smokers than in non-smokers of the same age. Although the exact relationship between cigarette smoking and osteoporosis is still being studied, research has revealed several ways smoking has an adverse affect on healthy bone mass:

■ Smokers are generally thinner than non-smokers, and thus probably have a lower percentage of body fat. Thin individuals have an increased risk for two reasons: First, there is less demand on the bones to support body weight, resulting in lower bone density than if the person did not smoke. In addition, fat tissue assists in the production of estrogen, and estrogen helps maintain bone mass.

■ Smoking may result in a woman's experiencing menopause earlier (some experts estimate up to five years earlier) than she would have had she not smoked. Early menopause translates to an increased risk for osteoporosis due to loss of the estrogen produced by the ovaries: The greater the number of years without estrogen, the greater the amount of bone loss over a lifetime. In addition, smoking results in the liver's changing estrogen into a compound that is less usable in building bone.

■ Smoking affects the processing of vitamin D, resulting in less calcium being absorbed by the system. Since calcium is critical to the mineralization, or hardening, phase of bone remodeling, inadequate levels of these nutrients drastically affect bone mass.

■ Smoking interferes with the normal production and use of the male hormone *testosterone*, increasing the risk of osteoporosis for men who smoke.

All smokers, *especially* those who have inherited risk factors for osteoporosis, are strongly urged to seek help to stop smoking.

SEDENTARY LIFESTYLE   It's safe to say that the days of lying on the sofa watching television while munching potato chips — *without* feeling guilty — are pretty much a thing of the past. The benefits of regular exercise as part of a healthy lifestyle have been well documented: Exercise has a positive effect on your heart, your weight and your overall sense of well-being. And now it's been proven that exercise has a significant beneficial effect on the condition of your bones.

Experts know that a lifestyle completely lacking in exercise (such as being bedridden for an extended period of time, or being weightless in space) results in significant loss of bone mass. In contrast, individuals who participate in a program of regular physical exercise benefit by a **decrease in the loss of bone mass**. Bones respond to physical demands by becoming more dense, thus stronger and less susceptible to fracture.

The exact extent of the benefits to bone mass from exercise are being researched. The leading authorities on this subject, however, consider exercise an integral part of any program for the treatment and prevention of osteoporosis.

EMOTIONAL STRESS   In today's fast-paced world, with so many demands for our time and attention, emotional and mental stress can be difficult to avoid. Not only is stress hard on your overall outlook, it has a negative impact on your skeletal system, as well. Stress increases the release of adrenal hormones. Since these hormones stimulate the cells that break down bone tissue, the body can lose bone mass. Stress also interferes with the absorption of calcium.

NO CHILDBEARING, OR HAVING AN ONLY CHILD THAT IS BREAST-FED   Pregnancy benefits bones in two ways: It elevates the levels of valuable hormones like estrogen, and it increases a woman's body weight for the period of pregnancy, both of which increase bone mass. While breast-feeding can drain calcium and other nutrients from the mother, this negative effect is offset by the positive effects of pregnancy if the mother bears more than one child.

The foods you eat have a direct effect on bone health, both positive and negative:

LACK OF CALCIUM   Calcium and its partner, vitamin D, are vital nutrients in the bone building process. Crystals of *calcium phosphate* compose much of the mass in bone tissue, and are the building blocks in the hardening phase of new bone formation. Without adequate calcium, bone cannot reach its maximum density and mass. The lower the bone density we accumulate in the first two to three decades of life, the more likely we are to become osteoporotic in later years.

As the body ages, its efficiency in absorbing and processing calcium decreases. If extra calcium is not available through the diet, the body may begin to rob the bones of calcium in order to put more of this vital nutrient into the bloodstream, where it is needed for normal muscle and nerve function, the proper clotting of blood and regulating the heartbeat. The result: loss of bone mass.

Studies indicate that a substantial percentage of women (who by virtue of their gender are already at risk for osteoporosis) get *less than half the calcium* they need every day. Other research shows that supplemental calcium may significantly reduce the risk of fractures. In fact, studies indicate that taking more calcium than the recommended daily allowance (RDA) can cut the risk of fracture by 60 percent or more.

Many different aspects of ordinary life can affect the body's absorption and processing of calcium, vitamin D and trace minerals such as boron, essential for bone building. Some of these are foods and drinks, such as caffeinated or alcoholic beverages and foods high in salt or phosphorus. Another factor is how we live our life: Emotional stress can increase the amount of calcium lost through urine; kidney disease has the same effect. Even a lack of sunshine can keep your body from processing calcium as it should: The body needs vitamin D to metabolize calcium, and sunshine is one source of vitamin D.

Some individuals experience *lactose intolerance.* Their bodies do not process milk products effectively, resulting in diarrhea and other intestinal problems. Anyone with this condition has a greater risk of osteoporosis if care is not taken to increase calcium in the diet from non-dairy sources, such as supplements.

The effects of dietary calcium on osteoporosis are explored more fully in Chapter Eight.

HIGH FIBER   While insoluble fiber, such as bran, has a positive effect on the digestive system and blood cholesterol, it can interfere with the body's ability to absorb calcium. No one recommends that you do away with fiber in your diet, but be aware that calcium binds with fiber and thus takes the "express train" out of your digestive system before it can be fully absorbed. Nutritionists suggest that you avoid combining high-fiber foods with calcium-rich foods in the same meal. Be especially conscious of taking adequate calcium if you're on a strict vegetarian diet. Fiber is a concern primarily for those who include little or no calcium in a high-fiber diet.

MEAT   A number of studies have linked excessive meat consumption to greater bone loss. Meat increases the loss of calcium through the kidneys. It is acidic, causing the body to use calcium to buffer the acids. This process depletes the calcium available to maintain healthy bones. Red meat also contains phosphorus, which in excessive amounts facilitates the loss of calcium. Many nutritionists suggest that a healthy overall diet include only three to six ounces of meat a day.

CARBONATED BEVERAGES   These popular drinks contain phosphorus in the form of phosphate, which naturally binds with calcium in the intestines, reducing its absorption. Some soft drinks contain caffeine and phosphoric acid, which also decrease calcium absorption.

EXCESS SALT   For women, especially during and after menopause, too much salt in the diet can lead to needed calcium being excreted through the urine.

Below and on the following page you will find a short quiz that can help you identify both inherited and lifestyle factors that increase your risk for osteoporosis. You are urged to discuss *all* of the risk factors that pertain to you with your medical professional, and get an expert's opinion on how you can best minimize your risk of osteoporosis.

Osteoporosis: Are You at Risk?

Check the box that best answers each question. Each "Yes" box with a check reflects an increase in your overall risk of osteoporosis.

YES   NO

❏   ❏   1. Are you female?

❏   ❏   2. Have you stopped menstruating?

❏   ❏   3. Is your heritage Caucasian or Oriental?

❏   ❏   4. Are you thin or small-boned, or do you have a low percentage of body fat?

❏   ❏   5. Does anyone in your family have a history of osteoporosis, especially bone fractures in older female relatives?

YES   NO

❑   ❑   6.   Did you start menopause before age 45?

❑   ❑   7.   Do you drink three or more alcoholic or caffeinated beverages a day?

❑   ❑   8.   Do you now smoke, or have you smoked in the past?

❑   ❑   9.   Do you lead a sedentary or physically inactive lifestyle?

❑   ❑   10. Do you rarely drink milk or eat dairy products?

❑   ❑   11. Is your diet high in salt, or in red meat or other animal proteins, or are you a strict vegetarian?

❑   ❑   12. Have you taken medication on a continuing basis for any of these conditions or diseases?

____ Thyroid disease

____ Asthma

____ Arthritis

____ Kidney or liver disease

____ Cancer

____ Diabetes

CHAPTER 4

Osteoporosis Screening and Diagnosis

From the time we are born our bodies are poked, prodded, pinched and pricked in an effort to assure our continued good health. And in most cases, rightly so. Infants and children, especially, are routinely screened for diseases and conditions that can be life-threatening, with widespread testing leading to significant decreases in such diseases as tuberculosis.

Children make up only one part of the population undergoing routine medical testing. Most menstruating women see a gynecologist each year for a Papanicolaou test — commonly called a *pap smear* — aimed at the early detection of uterine and cervical cancer. The number of women undergoing mammograms to detect breast cancer is steadily increasing. Almost all pregnant women are tested for gestational diabetes, and those over 35 often have sonograms and amniocentesis in an effort to ensure a healthy newborn. And, as a sign of our times, more men and women are having themselves tested for HIV, the virus that causes AIDS, with a clean bill of health sometimes presented as a "rite of passage" from a romantic involvement into a sexual relationship.

In the world of medicine, a test may be performed on a patient for one of two reasons: *screening* or *diagnosis.* In layperson's terms, a screening test is one that is recommended for a person who is part of a group especially susceptible to a disease or condition, but who does not show any outward symptoms. The mammogram, used to detect breast cancer in its early stages, is a good example of a screening test: Though a woman may not exhibit symptoms of breast cancer, if she is over 40 years old and has a family history of the disease, she is part of a group at increased risk of developing breast cancer. Thus she is a good candidate for the test that screens for the disease.

A diagnostic test, on the other hand, is performed when a patient shows symptoms of a disease or condition. The physician seeks to verify a diagnosis, rule out secondary causes of the symptoms and determine the extent of damage or disease. The test method used for screening might also be used for diagnosis; the difference is not in the test itself, but in the reason the test is given and how the results are used.

This chapter discusses the differences between a screening test and a diagnostic test for osteoporosis, and what the tests are looking for. It airs both sides of the medical debate over the value of screening women for osteoporosis, and introduces the medical specialties that commonly treat the disease. It covers the most popular methods of testing for osteoporosis, the advantages and disadvantages of each, and what to expect when you undergo a screening or diagnostic test.

What the Tests Measure: How Healthy Are Your Bones?

Recent advances in technology have provided significant improvements in detecting bone loss. Your doctor will use one of several *bone density tests* that are currently available. These tests measure the level of bone density at selected sites in the skeleton, and allow the doctor to compare your measurement to the average for non-osteoporotic women your age.

Learning the Lingo

Bone Mineral Content (BMC): The amount of calcium and other trace minerals in bone tissue, it is expressed in terms of grams (of mineral) per square centimeter (of bone). BMC correlates directly to the density of bone: the higher the bone mineral content, the denser the bones.

Fracture Threshold: In interpreting screening and diagnostic test results, the fracture threshold refers to a bone mineral content that correlates to a fracture rate *two times* higher than that of a non-osteoporotic person. The fracture threshold marks the boundary between low bone density and actual osteoporosis.

Doctors refer to bone density in terms of *bone mineral content*. The terms bone density and bone mineral content are often used interchangeably. Both refer to the amount of hardened calcium phosphate in the bones. This substance is deposited in bone during the mineralization phase of bone remodeling. These mineral crystals are lost when bone tissue is broken down during the resorption phase of the remodeling process. If the bone destroyer cells are breaking down more bone than can be replaced by the bone builder cells, your body is using these minerals without replacing them. The result is a steady decrease in bone density, referred to simply as *bone loss.*

Researchers have determined that when bone mineral content falls below a certain point, bones become extremely prone to fracture. This point of impending injury is called the *fracture threshold.* If your test reveals low bone density but your bone mineral content has not yet reached the fracture threshold, you have a condition called *osteopenia.* Osteopenia is the precursor to osteoporosis, because if bones continue to lose density, they will eventually reach the fracture threshold. If your test shows that your bone mineral content is below the fracture threshold, you have *osteoporosis.* These classifications are often ignored, with low bone density in general referred to as osteoporosis.

Screening for Osteoporosis

The purpose of a *screening test* for osteoporosis is to determine the patient's current bone mineral content, and to develop a bone maintenance program that will help prevent bone density from reaching the fracture threshold. A screening test for osteoporosis can also predict the likelihood that a person will develop the disease.

Your doctor may recommend a screening test if you meet certain conditions that put you at risk for low bone density. Some of the criteria include your sex and age, the status of your reproductive system (whether you are postmenopausal or have had a hysterectomy) and whether you have been on long-term therapy with one of several drugs known to accelerate bone loss.

Most of us rely on the advice of our doctors to determine which tests we should undergo. But how does your doctor determine which patients need testing? Some doctors will use a short quiz for risk factors, like the one in Chapter Three; others may routinely recommend screening tests for all women around the age of menopause; still other physicians may not recommend screening at all, leaving it to the patient to broach the subject.

The Screening Controversy

The method — or lack of method — for selecting women to be screened for osteoporosis is a matter of some debate within the medical community. There is a wide difference of opinion concerning which women need to be screened: On one side of the issue are doctors who feel that *all* postmenopausal women should be tested for low bone density, while other doctors feel that only those women who show indications of known risks should be screened. From a financial point of view, the group that advocates screening all postmenopausal women claims that such blanket testing would be cost-effective. They say that the expense of screening would be offset by the savings to individuals and to society in treating far fewer complications of osteoporotic fractures. Those who disagree with blanket screening fear it will be misused for financial gain within the medical community, and that screening is an unnecessary expense for some patients.

Cost is just one argument in this issue. General screening criteria for osteoporosis would have far-reaching impact, not only financially, but physically and emotionally, as well. At a meeting of the National Osteoporosis Foundation in 1990, a task force presented data concluding that as many as 750,000 bone fractures in postmenopausal women could be prevented *each year* with properly applied screening criteria and the new detection methods. Millions of Americans — the aging baby boomers — are approaching the age that puts them at increased risk for osteoporosis, and billions of dollars and many, many lives hang in the balance.

Screening Tests and Health Insurance

Major health insurers have begun to recognize the value of preventive care in general. In 1991, the largest health insurance company in America, Blue Cross and Blue Shield, announced a preventive care program that includes screening tests for certain diseases. The company published a schedule recommending who should have the tests and at what age they should be tested. Osteoporosis is one of the diseases included in this preventive care program, along with heart disease, diabetes, and cancer of the lung, colon, breast and cervix. The Blue Cross and Blue Shield preventive care program is not yet available to policyholders nationwide, but insurance industry experts feel that most private insurers will follow suit. They cite the fact that preventive care makes good economic sense for the insurance companies, for the country and for *you.*

For those Americans who are over age 65, the policies of *Medicare* may dictate whether they receive preventive health care. Medicare is health insurance for people over 65, and some younger disabled people. Although Medicare is funded by the federal government, Medicare dollars are turned over to individual states to administer. Your state, in turn, decides which medical tests and procedures it will cover, and the amount that it will pay for these services. Coverages vary widely from state to state: In one state, Medicare pays up to $120 for an osteoporosis screening test, while a nearby state pays only $70 for the same test. Some states will not pay for osteoporosis screening tests at all. The best way to find out what Medicare will pay where you live is to start with a call to your doctor's office, since the staff is usually aware of what is covered. If you want additional information about Medicare, call your local Social Security office, listed in the government section of the telephone directory.

Though osteoporosis is certainly not a new condition, it has only recently become a health issue of significant focus. Now that the big insurance powers recognize the disease as an economic threat and have begun to pay for preventive care, one would expect that the medical community will become more sensitive to osteoporosis and will be more apt to recommend routine screening. **Ultimately, however, it is your responsibility to initiate a discussion about osteoporosis screening with your doctor.**

Should You Be Screened for Osteoporosis?

A medical test is but one tool in a complete health care program. Before deciding whether a test is warranted for a particular patient, a doctor must weigh many factors, not the least of which should be the wants and needs of the patient. Controversy has arisen in recent years concerning physicians who schedule unnecessary tests for their patients. In some cases, these doctors were affiliated with a testing or diagnostic center and recommended unneeded tests to reap personal financial profits. Other physicians — because of the "take 'em to court" attitude of our society — schedule tests that they honestly do not believe are necessary, as protection against malpractice suits.

Bear in mind your goal in reading this book: to educate yourself about osteoporosis. Why not apply to *yourself* some of the standards that medical professionals use to determine whether a test is warranted? Ultimately, *you* are responsible for your own health. Asking yourself and your doctor these questions may help you decide whether you want to be screened for osteoporosis:

■ The test itself must return accurate results. How trustworthy is the data for predicting risk?

■ What is the risk of injury, side effect or discomfort from the testing procedure? How does this balance with the danger of injury if I am not tested?

■ If the test indicates that I am at risk, can the condition be effectively treated, or can I diminish my chances of developing the disease?

■ What is the cost of the test? Is it within my means to pay, or does my insurance cover it?

An important point to remember: The presence of osteoporosis risk factors does not accurately predict *fractures*. A woman with many risk factors may never suffer an osteoporotic fracture, while a woman with few risk factors may suffer repeated fractures. Along the same lines, a risk factor quiz or a single screening test cannot accurately predict the *rate* at which anyone will lose bone mass — diet, exercise, illness, medication and lifestyle are in a state of constant change. A woman who is not at apparent risk at age 50 may be osteoporotic at age 60.

National Osteoporosis Foundation Guidelines for Clinical Bone Mass Measurement

Bone mass measurement is justified:

■ To provide information on bone density to estrogen-deficient women who are faced with a decision on whether to undergo hormone replacement therapy.

■ To confirm a diagnosis of spinal osteoporosis and to evaluate treatment options for patients with vertebral abnormalities or low bone mass detected by standard X-ray.

■ To diagnose low bone mass and evaluate therapy options for patients who have been on a long-term program of medication with drugs known to contribute to bone loss.

■ To diagnose low bone mass in patients with overactive parathyroid glands, called **primary hyperparathyroidism**, and to help determine if the potential damage to the skeletal system warrants surgery, since most cases of hyperparathyroidism are caused by benign tumors.

A woman who is screened for osteoporosis will have the benefit of knowing where she stands when compared to the average or mean bone mass level for women her age. Screening for osteoporosis is usually not a one-shot deal, however. Even a woman with an average level of bone mass for her age should be retested to monitor her *personal* rate of bone loss. A woman's own rate of bone loss is the most accurate predictor of whether she is at risk of fractures from osteoporosis. How often a woman should be retested depends on her current bone density, her risk level and her age. Some experts retest their menopausal patients every six months, due to the rapid rate of bone loss in the years immediately following menopause. Women who are not at such high risk should be retested about once a year.

Robert Lang, M.D., is the Medical Director of the Osteoporosis Diagnostic and Treatment Centers in New Haven and Bridgeport, Connecticut. Dr. Lang feels that frequent retesting of patients is crucial to avoiding fractures. "Testing a menopausal woman every six months allows you to identify those women who lose bone mass very rapidly, and to get started on early intervention."

The goal of a screening test is to detect the risk of osteoporosis at a point at which it is possible to initiate an effective prevention and treatment program that will help reduce the risk of future fractures.

The same bone density test may be used for both screening and diagnosis, but physicians sometimes use a slightly different technique when screening for osteoporosis. One such technique is referred to as a "quick pass" or "rapid measurement," which indicates overall bone density. If the results of this test indicate low bone density, the physician may advise that the patient undergo a more thorough bone density measurement, such as the techniques used for diagnostic purposes.

Armed with the knowledge of her current bone density and her rate of bone loss, a woman can make informed decisions about her diet, exercise program and controversial health issues such as estrogen replacement therapy. In addition, many doctors feel that patients who have been screened for osteoporosis are more aware of the impact that diet, exercise and estrogen have on bone mass, and that aware women are more apt to stick with the long-term commitment necessary in the effective treatment of osteoporosis.

Should you and your doctor decide that a screening test for osteoporosis is appropriate, you can expect to be given one or more of the most common bone density tests. A description of these tests begins on page 60.

Diagnosing Osteoporosis

A *diagnostic test* for osteoporosis is performed on a person who shows symptoms of the disease. Physical indications of osteoporosis can be a sudden intense pain, a spontaneous fracture, loss of height or a "dowager's hump," the telltale bent-forward posture that strongly indicates previous vertebral fractures. A physician will usually recommend a bone density test as a means of confirming the diagnosis.

Many women who undergo a screening test will find out that they have osteoporosis, even though they have not yet experienced a fracture. If a screening test reveals that you have osteopenia or osteoporosis, in effect it becomes a diagnostic test. This can be an important distinction in whether or not the test is covered by insurance, and your doctor should note the results on the proper forms.

As you can see, the line separating screening tests and diagnostic tests is blurred when it comes to osteoporosis. This is primarily because of the huge number of women who develop the condition,

Osteoporosis Warning Signs

 hile it is never too early to talk to your doctor about osteoporosis, it is essential that you bring up the subject if:

■ You experience sudden intense pain, especially in the spine, hip or wrist, that does not respond to over-the-counter pain medication.

■ You notice symptoms that may indicate decreasing levels of estrogen or the onset of menopause, such as irregular or infrequent menstrual periods, night sweats, fatigue, hot flashes and mood swings.

and because screening has not been as widely available in the past. Since as many as half of all women over the age of 50 will eventually suffer a bone fracture due to osteoporosis, a doctor who *screens* all post-menopausal patients will actually *diagnose* the disease in as many as 50 percent of those women.

For a woman who has not had a screening test to detect low bone density, a sudden acute pain — most often in the lower back — that does not respond to over-the-counter pain medication may be the first indication that she suffers from osteoporosis. What can a woman expect upon visiting her doctor for such a symptom? The doctor will first try to determine whether osteoporosis is a factor by asking questions about her medical history, looking for any medications, lifestyle factors or family history that would indicate she is at risk. Next may come a physical examination, with the doctor looking for changes, such as a loss of height, that can point to osteoporosis. The doctor will then probably schedule an *X-ray* of the painful area, the first in what may be a series of tests.

Should the X-ray indeed reveal a vertebral fracture, the doctor will want to determine whether osteoporosis is definitely at fault. Along with one or more of the bone density tests, the doctor may also take urine and blood samples that will be used to check

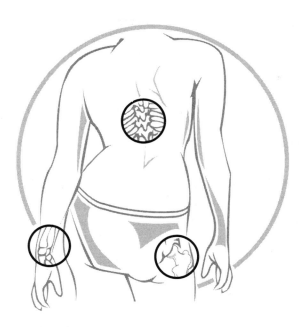

Bone fractures due to osteoporosis occur most often in the wrist, hip and spine. Of the more than 1.3 million osteoporotic fractures that occur each year in the United States, about 250,000 are fractures of the hip. Nearly 50,000 Americans die each year as a result of complications from a hip fracture.

**Most common sites for osteoporotic fractures:
Wrist, spine, hip**

important metabolic indicators that reveal how well the body is remodeling bone and the remodeling rate.

While the fracture itself may point to a diagnosis of osteoporosis, tests can determine to what extent the patient has suffered bone loss, in addition to confirming the presence of the disorder. Patients who experience an osteoporotic fracture of the spine are about four times as likely also to fracture a hip. Doctors often use diagnostic testing after an initial injury to determine the amount of bone loss in other sites at high risk for fractures (the hip, spine and wrist being the top three). Bone density measurements and laboratory tests are also used to rule out secondary causes of fractures, such as other bone diseases. These tests are also given to previously diagnosed patients to determine whether they are responding well to treatment.

Specialists Who Treat Osteoporosis

If you are diagnosed with low bone density or osteoporosis, your first objective may be to find the finest specialist available to help you manage the condition. While a number of medical specialties treat patients with osteoporosis, there is no single medical specialty that is dedicated solely to the diagnosis and treatment of that disease. The best place to begin your search is with your family doctor or gynecologist, who should be aware of physicians in your area who are actively involved in osteoporosis treatment.

This is not to say that your own doctor cannot guide you in the prevention and treatment of osteoporosis, but there are physicians who have devoted the bulk of their practice to treating osteoporotic patients. Most doctors regularly attend medical seminars and conferences to keep current on those issues directly affecting their own patients. The doctors in your area who treat a significant number of osteoporosis patients are therefore most likely to be up-to-date on the newest prevention, treatment and diagnostic methods.

A number of large hospitals and university medical centers have departments dedicated to the study, diagnosis and treatment of osteoporosis. At these facilities you are most likely to find state-of-the-art diagnostic machinery and the latest in new or experimental osteoporosis treatment programs. In addition, large hospitals increasingly offer organized support groups or workshops for individuals suffering from osteoporosis. Read the appendix for more information on these resources; workshops and support groups offer a wealth of useful information and can help steer you to those physicians in your area who stay current on new treatment programs for osteoporosis.

The medical specialists who most commonly treat osteoporosis include the following, in alphabetical order:

Endocrinologists   These are doctors who diagnose and treat diseases and disorders of the glands, called the endocrine system. The hormones produced by the glands play an important role in building and maintaining healthy bones.

Family Practice Physicians   These doctors are probably most familiar with you and your medical history. Most have experience in internal medicine and gynecology, and some surgical training.

Geriatricians   These doctors specialize in the treatment of elderly patients. Most are family practice physicians or internists who have received additional training in the diseases associated with aging.

Gynecologists   Specialists in the female reproductive system, these physicians often provide a woman with her first information on osteoporosis as part of a discussion on the effects of menopause. Gynecologists are the specialists most likely to discuss estrogen replacement therapy and the effect it has on bone mass. Most gyne-cologists also perform surgery on the female reproductive system. Some of these doctors are OB/GYNs. The OB stands for *obstetrics*, which encompasses the treatment of pregnant women and the delivery of babies.

Internists   Sometimes referred to as internal medicine doctors, these physicians treat diseases and conditions of the entire body, but do not perform surgery.

Orthopedic Surgeons   These physicians diagnose and treat disorders of the musculoskeletal system, which includes the muscles and bones. Injuries to bones and joints are typically treated by these doctors, who rely heavily on surgical techniques.

Rheumatologists   These are internists who have received addi-tional training in the diagnosis and treatment of disorders of the joints, muscles and bones. They commonly treat disorders such as arthritis and lupus, as well as osteoporosis. Rheumatologists, as a rule, do not perform surgery.

Searching Out Osteoporosis: Bone Density Measurement

Several testing methods are commonly used to analyze bone density. Naming just one of these methods as the best for identifying fracture risk is a matter of some debate within the medical community. Each of the tests has advantages and disadvantages, but being tested for osteoporosis using *any* of them is preferable to not being tested at all.

A bone density test measures how strong the bones are by determining the bone mineral content of one or more sites in the skeleton. The most commonly tested sites include the heel, the forearm, the spine and the hip; some tests can measure the total bone mass of the entire skeleton. Do not confuse bone density measurement with a **bone scan,** in which an isotope is injected to help detect diseases of the bone, such as cancer.

A standard X-ray cannot detect bone loss until 25 to 40 percent of bone mass is lost. The techniques used in bone density measurement are much more precise. All of the bone density tests described here utilize the science of **radiology.** They use either radioactive elements called **isotopes** or an X-ray source to provide radiation. The radiation exposure from the testing machines called **absorptiometers** is very limited; they emit levels that are less than that of a standard chest X-ray. The **Quantitative Computed Tomography** (**QCT** or **CAT scan**) emits a great deal more energy.

In each bone density test, one or more streams of radiant energy are projected through the skeletal test site. The machine calculates the amount of energy absorbed by the bone to determine bone mineral content. The more energy absorbed, the denser the bone.

The data is sent to a computer that analyzes the information and prepares the test results. Your results will probably be presented in a graph format that illustrates your level of bone mineral content compared to that of an average non-osteoporotic woman your age. After you have a second bone density measurement, usually six months or a year later, your doctor can project, with some accuracy, your *rate* of bone loss. This allows you and the doctor to monitor and "fine tune" your prevention or treatment program, introducing alternate treatment methods if the test results show them to be necessary.

Which Bone Density Test Is Best?

By this point you may wonder which of the tests is best for you. In fact, the four most common bone density measurement tests are similar in technique, but differ in precision and accuracy. While all of the tests are acceptable for screening purposes, some do not have the precision necessary for follow-up testing, in which an accurate comparison to previous measurements is needed to evaluate the rate of bone loss. The primary differences between the tests lie in which skeletal sites and which types of bone (trabecular or cortical) they can most accurately measure.

Trabecular bone, the soft spongy bone that makes up much of the spine, is a metabolically active form of bone. This means it is more susceptible to rapid loss in response to changing conditions in the body (such as menopause). Because of this, many osteoporosis experts feel that a bone density test must be able to accurately measure trabecular bone, which not all of the tests can do. Some experts feel that measurement of the bone mineral content of the heel bone (*os calcis*) can accurately indicate trabecular bone density throughout the skeleton. This is called single-site measurement. Its advocates also believe that measurement of a forearm bone (*radius*) is an effective means of assessing cortical bone density throughout the body. Opponents of the single-site concept feel that a direct correlation has not been firmly established between bone density measurements of the heel and forearm and the actual density of the spine or hip.

Everyone agrees, however, that measurement of all three primary osteoporotic fracture sites (wrist, spine and hip) is the optimum choice if the technology is available in your area and you and your doctor feel the cost is justified. For now, naming one or two skeletal sites as the best indicators of fracture risk needs further research.

Each of the bone density tests has its proponents and its advantages. In conjunction with your doctor, you must first determine which tests are available in your area. Then, consider the following factors in choosing a test method:

- How detailed do my results need to be? Can a single-site measurement that estimates overall bone mass provide me with enough information?

- Do I have risk factors (such as heredity or age) that indicate I am at significant risk for osteoporosis, and should look into one of the more comprehensive tests?

- What is the difference in my cost of the available tests in my area?

The statistics are alarming: There is a significant association between hip fracture and loss of life or independence. Anyone who has been diagnosed with osteoporosis should seriously consider undergoing one of the tests that directly measure the primary fracture sites. Make certain that you and your doctor agree that whatever test you select will provide you with the information you need to make informed decisions about your particular state of health.

C. Conrad Johnston, Jr., M.D., is Professor of Medicine and Director of the Division of Endocrinology and Metabolism at Indiana University Medical Center. "Bone mass measurements are the best method of identifying persons at risk for fracture," he says. "If you want to assess an individual's *overall* fracture risk, then all of the bone mass measurement techniques are about equal in effectiveness. To estimate the fracture risk of a certain site, however, it is best to use a method that *accurately* measures that site. If an individual's greatest concern is a hip fracture, then it is best to measure the hip."

Not all diagnostic facilities, whether they be hospitals, doctors' offices or diagnostic centers, have the equipment for testing all three of the common fracture sites. As you will see in the discussion of each method, only a couple of the bone density tests can measure *all* of those sites with significant accuracy. Remember, though, that even testing a single site is better than not being tested at all, as long as you are willing to follow a preventive or treatment program that includes exercise and proper diet, with the possibility of hormone therapy and medication.

Costs and Health Insurance

The four most widely available bone density tests vary in cost. What you pay in your city can be substantially more or less than the price of the same test in a different geographic area. To give you an idea of how significant this difference can be: One diagnostic center in the Northeast commonly charges about $300 to measure the density of

Bone Measurement Interpretive Report

Exam Date: 12/01/92
Patient: Jane Doe
Age: 65.4   Race: Caucasian   Sex: Female
Facility: The Women's Health Center
Physician: Richard Roe, M.D.
Bone site tested: Os calcis (heel) (95% trabecular bone)
BMC: 0.356 g/cm^2
Annual percent of change: +10.23% (two measurements required)

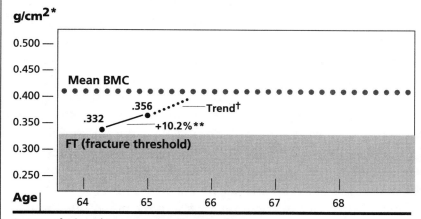

*grams of mineral per square centimeter of bone

** Annual rate of change.

† Projected trend is an average of the last two or three exams. (The projected BMC value is not necessarily predictive of actual BMC change.)

This graph is very similar to the one that you will review with your doctor after a bone density test. At the time of her first test, this 65-year-old patient's bone mineral content (BMC) was significantly below that of a non-osteoporotic woman her age (shown by the dotted line), and was dangerously close to the fracture threshold. The second test revealed that her bone mineral content had increased slightly, no doubt due to a treatment program developed in partnership with her physician after the first test. Note that the projected trend would continue to take her further from the fracture threshold. This projection assumes that all the factors that led to the increase in bone mineral content will remain constant: that she will continue to respond to the treatment and that no secondary factors contributing to bone loss — such as disease, or an illness or injury that requires extensive bed rest — will arise. However, a projected trend cannot predict exact future bone mineral content.

all three primary fracture sites with state-of-the-art technology; at another facility less than 30 miles away, the same test on the same skeletal sites costs about $450.

Insurance coverage for bone density tests is unpredictable. Some insurance companies pay for a diagnostic test but not one given for screening purposes, while other companies pay for screening tests in one state but not in another. Medicare also shows a wide variance in coverage: In Florida, Medicare pays about $120 for a bone density test, while Medicare in Louisiana pays only $70 for the same test. The best advice: Check with your insurance company *before* scheduling a test to avoid unpleasant surprises when filing a claim. If you are over age 65 or disabled and are on Medicare, be sure to talk to your doctor's staff or call your local Social Security office to find out whether these tests are covered and what your co-payment will be.

B. Lawrence Riggs, M.D., professor of Medical Research at Mayo Medical School and Director of the General Clinical Research Center at the Mayo Clinic in Rochester, Minnesota, indicates that participation by private insurers and Medicare plays a great role in the state of preventive health care for American women. "Standard screening criteria for osteoporosis are not in the immediate future because of the reimbursement issue. I believe that at some point in the future we will have standard reimbursement for screening, but we must first get the cost of the measurements down. I don't think we are too far off from a $50 rapid measurement that will determine whether you have low overall bone density."

What to Expect on Test Day

It is very likely that you will be sent to a hospital or other large diagnostic facility for your bone density test, because few doctors have the equipment for measuring bone density in their offices. As with many medical tests, a technician will take the measurements and pass along the results to your doctor. The doctor will usually schedule a follow-up visit to discuss the results of your test and to help you set up a bone maintenance or treatment program.

Before or after the test is done (usually not the same day), your doctor or a member of the staff may ask you about your medical history, family history (especially whether older relatives have experienced fractures) and lifestyle choices that may contribute to osteoporosis. Next will come a brief physical examination, with the doctor looking for physical indications of osteoporosis such as a decrease in height or abnormalities of the vertebrae.

No need to feel squeamish on test day — all four of the most widely available bone density tests are non-invasive, meaning that the body is not penetrated in any way during testing. Be advised, though, that you may be asked for both urine and blood samples during your visit. Several tests done with these bodily fluids reveal a great deal about how your body is performing the bone remodeling process.

Undergoing a Bone Density Test

All of the bone density tests work in a similar way. As discussed earlier, they direct one or more streams of radiant energy at the skeletal site to be measured, with the energy streams passing through the bone and surrounding soft tissues. The machine measures how much radiation passes through the bone. The denser the bone, the smaller the amount of radiation that will pass through it; the rest is absorbed by the bone. The machine calculates bone mineral content based on the amount of radiation that was absorbed by the bone.

If you undergo a test that measures the bone mineral content of the heel or forearm, you will be in a seated position. The heel or forearm will rest on a surface that is shaped to accommodate it.

If your spine or hip is measured you will lie atop a scanner table. The energy source will be beneath you, while the mechanism that counts the amount of radiation passing through the bone will be positioned above the table. You may be asked to bend your knees while your spine is measured, so that the lower back presses against the table.

The technique of quantitative computed tomography (CAT scan) is different from the tests that use an absorptiometer. This test is most often used to measure the vertebrae; the patient lies on her back on a table and is moved into a large cylindrical tube, somewhat resembling a tunnel. As with the other tests, radiation is projected through the bone and soft tissues.

The procedure is over fairly quickly, with the newer machines completing the actual testing in just a few minutes. You should experience little or no discomfort during any of the bone density measurements. Keep in mind that the time estimates given in the test descriptions are the time it takes to do the bone measurements, not the total amount of time required for your visit to the testing center.

The Four Most Common Bone Density Tests

Although the tests are similar in technique and function, they differ substantially in the type of bone and the skeletal site that they can accurately measure. Listed are the four most widely available methods of bone density measurement, beginning with the original technology and moving on to the machines that are currently considered state-of-the-art.

Single Photon Absorptiometry (SPA)

Test Site   Forearm bone (radius) and heel (os calcis).

Comments   Developed in the 1960s, Single Photon Absorptiometry was the first method of bone density measurement, and remains the most widely available. It uses a single beam of radiation, making it unable to distinguish between soft tissue (like organs) and bone. This limitation restricts SPA to use on the limbs.

Proponents of this technique feel that measurement of bone mineral content in the heel is an accurate indicator of trabecular bone density throughout the skeleton, with the forearm bone performing the same function for cortical bone throughout the body.

Advantages   Can be done quickly; measurements are completed in about 10 minutes. Medicare pays in most states.

Disadvantages   Cannot test spine and hips. Cannot distinguish between bone and soft tissue, nor can it distinguish trabecular bone from cortical bone.

Dual Photon Absorptiometry (DPA)

Test Site   Hip and spine.

Comments   First developed in the early 1980s, DPA uses radioactive sources (radioisotopes) that project two streams of radiant energy through the test areas. This allows DPA to accurately distinguish bone from soft tissue, so it can be used on the hip and spine where the radiation must pass through the body cavity or organs. Measurements take about 20 or 30 minutes.

Advantages   Better than Single Photon Absorptiometry for measuring bone mineral content and assessing fracture risk of spine and hip. Can also measure total skeletal bone mass.

Disadvantages   DPA cannot distinguish between cortical and trabecular bone. It is not readily available in all areas. DPA is not sensitive enough to use for follow-up tests. May be considered experimental technology by some insurance companies and Medicare, and thus not covered.

Quantitative Computed Tomography (QCT, commonly called CAT scan)

Test Site   Can test all areas, but most commonly used on spine.

Comments   This test is quite flexible, although experts differ in opinion on the accuracy of its measurement. QCT can provide separate measurement of cortical and trabecular bone, or a combined total bone mass. The results can be produced as a three-dimensional image of the scanned area. Measurement of the spine usually takes about 20 minutes.

Advantages   Allows testing of all types and locations of bone; especially beneficial in measuring bone mineral content of trabecular bone in the spine.

Disadvantages   Highest levels of radiation; can exceed 100 times the radiation dose of DPA and DEXA. QCT is quite expensive, costing several hundred dollars or more.

Dual X-Ray (or Dual Energy) Absorptiometry (DEXA)

Test Site   Hip, spine and wrist.

Comments   Developed in the late 1980s, DEXA is considered state-of-the-art technology. It is similar to Dual Photon Absorptiometry in technique, but it uses X-ray radiation. The X-rays are filtered into two levels of energy, allowing accurate measurement of the hip and spine, as well as the wrist.

Advantages   Lowest radiation dose. Quickest of the four tests — all three primary fracture sites can be measured in five or six minutes. Allows the most precise testing of both types of bone tissue, and provides high resolution images.

Disadvantages   Is not readily available in all areas. DEXA is more expensive than SPA and DPA.

"Dual energy X-ray absorptiometry is really the gold standard [in bone density measurement] now," says Dr. Lang. "It is highly accurate, the results are reproducible in follow-up tests, and it is very fast. With the newest technology we can measure all three primary fracture sites in less than five minutes. And as more machines become available, it will become less expensive."

In interviews with the experts, Dr. Lang's opinion was echoed time and time again. It seems unanimous among those in the know that dual energy X-ray absorptiometry is state-of-the-art. There are other techniques for bone density measurement in addition to the four described above, but they are not widely available and are not considered to be as accurate.

Blood and Urine Tests

At some point in your testing, the doctor will want to collect blood and urine samples. Blood and urine contain hormones, nutrients and other chemicals that are by-products of the body's metabolic processes. These substances are sometimes referred to as *biochemical markers*. The presence and amount of these biochemical markers in the blood or urine reveal a great deal about your overall health, as well as being significant indicators of how well your body is performing the bone remodeling process, and at what rate.

These tests are vital to assure your physician that there are no secondary factors — causes other than osteoporosis — contributing to bone loss. Secondary factors would include an undiagnosed disease or a hormonal imbalance. The tests also check whether your body is sufficiently able to metabolize, or make use of, the nutrients necessary to build and maintain healthy bones.

In the late 1980s, two tests were developed to measure biochemical markers in the blood that indicate the rate of ***bone turnover***. Bone turnover refers to the rate at which the body performs the remodeling process, destroying old bone and replacing it with new bone. At certain times during life, the blood will have elevated levels of these biochemical markers, indicating a high rate of bone turnover. During the teen years, this high rate is due to the accelerated skeletal growth occurring after puberty. In postmenopausal women, however, an elevated level of these biochemical markers indicates bone loss.

Experts believe that measuring bone density *and* testing blood and urine for bone-specific biomarkers is the future trend in assessing fracture risk. These experts are convinced that this combination will be much more effective in detecting and monitoring bone loss than using bone density tests alone.

Dr. Riggs says, "With the advances that have been made in bone densitometry, combined with the measurement of bone chemical markers, we are now very close to being able to identify the target population at greatest risk for osteoporosis and to intervene before fractures occur."

After the Testing: On the Road to Healthier Bones

After all the test results are in, you can anticipate another conversation with your doctor. This meeting may or may not take place on the day of your testing, depending on how your doctor handles the processing of the blood and urine tests.

If your screening test reveals average or higher bone mass, you should receive information on proper diet and exercise to maintain healthy bones. You may be asked to schedule another screening test to be performed in a year or so, depending on your bone density level in this test.

Common Bone-Related Urine and Blood Tests

Test	Indication	Source
Calcium-to-Creatinine Ratio	Evaluates the processing of calcium.	Urine
Hydroxyproline and Pyridinolines Levels	Measures biomarkers of bone turnover. Elevated levels indicate high rate of bone turnover.	Urine
Thyroid and Parathyroid Function	Indicates calcium levels in bloodstream; evaluates metabolic functions.	Blood
Osteocalcin Level	Provides indications of bone formation.	Blood
Malabsorption Tests	Checks that nutrients are being processed properly.	Blood
Hormone Levels	Measures follicle-stimulating hormone (FSH) in the bloodstream; elevated levels indicate estrogen deficiency. Also used to measure estrogen and testosterone levels.	Blood

If you are diagnosed with osteoporosis or significantly low bone density, your doctor will want to discuss your treatment options. A number of resources are available in the fight to hold on to bone mass. Some are familiar, like estrogen and calcium. Others, such as the substances used in drug therapy, are not as familiar, but may play an integral role in the combination of methods that will make up your osteoporosis treatment program.

The next four chapters focus on the four main components of an osteoporosis prevention and treatment program: **Hormone therapy, drug therapy, exercise and diet.**

CHAPTER 5

Hormones, Menopause and the Great Estrogen Debate

ormones are complex chemicals produced by glands and organs throughout the body. They are both the catalysts and the regulators of our most fundamental bodily functions, like heartbeat and digestion. From the time of conception, hormones have a profound effect on the minds and bodies of all human beings. Are you moody at certain times of the month? Have you ever experienced jet lag? Do some of your friends seem to get pregnant at the drop of a hat, while others may struggle for years to conceive a child? Have you noticed that some men have an abundance of body hair or a baritone voice, while others do not? If you have observed the unique characteristics that make one human being different from another, you have been touched by the effect that hormones have on all of us.

In many ways, the study of hormones and the organs and glands that produce them — called *endocrinology* — is still in its infancy. More than 200 hormones are known to be produced by the human body, and scientists are identifying others with surprising regularity. The profound impact that hormones have on the functioning of our bodies and on our behavior is under intense study throughout the world. The complex interrelationships among these powerful chemicals are of particular interest to many scientists. Researchers feel certain that solving some of our most serious health problems — cancer, heart disease, immune system disorders and osteoporosis, to name a few — depends on a greater understanding of our complicated hormonal network.

Hormones: Key Players in the Formation of Healthy Bones

With all its components working in harmony as they were designed to do, the human body is truly an awe-inspiring system of interaction on virtually every level. From the ways that different types of cells communicate, to the physical dexterity provided by muscles and bones working together, the body is a tribute to the concept of teamwork. Hormones play the part of team coach, sending signals that tell the body what to do and when to do it.

In order to understand the effect hormones have on the body, you must first understand that hormones have a profound effect on one another. The influence of the pituitary gland on human reproduction is a good example: Follicle-stimulating hormone produced by the pituitary gland stimulates the secretion of another hormone, estrogen, by the gonads. Estrogen, in turn, helps regulate the female menstrual cycle. Like good team players, the hormones within the endocrine system depend upon one another to accomplish such intricate tasks as reproduction, digestion, metabolism — and bone remodeling.

Hormones communicate by way of microscopic pathways, called *receptors*, that lie on the surface of cells or within them. Receptors are not open doors through which any body chemical from the bloodstream can enter. Only cells that have receptors for a particular hormone are directly affected by that hormone. Cells that have receptors for a specific hormone are referred to as being *responsive* to that hormone. Identifying which cells are responsive to which hormones is part of the challenge faced by researchers studying osteoporosis and other diseases.

Some glands, like the pituitary and thyroid, manufacture

hormones from protein. Other hormones are produced by glands on an "as needed" basis from cholesterol in the bloodstream. These hormones are called *steroids*. Estrogen, testosterone and the adrenal hormones are steroids, and so is one of the nutrients critical to healthy bone, *vitamin D*.

A major challenge faced by researchers is finding a way to intervene when specific hormone levels fall or rise. Too much or too little of one hormone can have a devastating effect on normal body functions — including bone remodeling.

Several glands in the endocrine system affect the bone remodeling process, but those producing hormones that play the most direct roles in bone formation and maintenance are:

Pituitary gland Found in the lower part of the brain, the pituitary gland has a significant effect on the function of other glands in the endocrine system, such as the adrenal and thyroid glands, as well as the gonads. Scientists have identified eight hormones produced by the pituitary gland itself, including *somatotropin*, which stimulates body growth, and *follicle-stimulating hormone*, which stimulates the secretion of the bone-friendly hormone, estrogen. Another pituitary hormone, *oxytocin*, stimulates contraction of the uterus during labor and childbirth, and causes milk to be released from the mammary glands during nursing. The pituitary gland has such great influence on other glands and on hormonal activity that it is sometimes referred to as the "master gland."

Hypothalamus A portion of the brain that lies at the base of the cerebrum, the hypothalamus indirectly controls much of the body's hormonal activity as a result of its effect on the pituitary gland. It plays a part in the regulation of body temperature, heart rate and blood pressure, the metabolism of fat and carbohydrates and the balance of body fluids.

Kidneys The kidneys not only filter water and remove waste products from the blood, they also produce enzymes and hormones that have a considerable effect on processes throughout the body. These hormones affect the levels of substances like potassium and calcium in the blood, and the activation of vitamin D.

Adrenal glands   There are two of these glands, one on top of each kidney. The adrenals produce in excess of 25 identified hormones, some of which contribute to bone loss. Each adrenal gland is divided into two parts. The *cortex* produces such hormones as the *glucocorticoids*, which regulate the amount of sugar in the blood, and *cortisone*, a hormone that helps the parathyroid hormones to stimulate the breakdown of bone. The cortex also produces *androgens*, the male sex hormones, in both men *and* women. The *medulla* produces a different set of hormones, including epinephrine, often called *adrenaline*, the "fight or flight" hormone produced in response to fear, anger or stress. Epinephrine has a dramatic effect on the body: It elevates the blood pressure, releases sugar from the liver to produce quick energy for the muscles and increases the heart rate.

Thyroid gland   Located in the neck, this gland produces two hormones that regulate the body's metabolic rate. *Metabolism* is the body's process of dispersing nutrients absorbed into the bloodstream as a result of digestion. It has two phases: *Anabolic* is the constructive phase, in which nutrient compounds are converted into more complex substances needed for normal functioning by the body cells. *Catabolic* is the destructive phase, in which the substances are broken back down into simple compounds, releasing energy for use by body cells.

In addition to the thyroid gland's function of regulating the body's metabolism, specialized cells in the thyroid gland produce a hormone called *calcitonin* when there is a high level of calcium in the blood. Calcitonin inhibits the breakdown of bone and is one of the primary drug treatments for osteoporosis.

Parathyroid glands   Found just behind the thyroid, these four tiny glands produce the hormones responsible for regulating the amount of calcium in the blood. The *parathyroid hormones* (PTH) play a key part in the bone remodeling process. When there is insufficient calcium in the blood, the parathyroid hormones stimulate the osteoclasts, the bone-destroying cells, to increase their activity, and the calcium stored within bone is released into the bloodstream. The blood calcium level then increases, and the parathyroid hormone has done its job.

Much of the focus of osteoporosis research is directed at repressing and controlling the destruction of bone put into motion by the parathyroid hormones.

Gonads This term refers to both the male and female sex glands. Everyone, male and female, produces small amounts of both types of sex hormones, though women generally have only a tiny percentage of male hormones, and vice versa.

In men, the *testes* manufacture male sex hormones called *androgens.* These hormones, such as *testosterone* and *androsterone,* are responsible for such male characteristics as heavy facial hair and a deep voice. Testosterone also has a protective effect on bone.

The *ovaries,* two walnut-sized glands located on each side of the uterus in the lower abdomen, produce the female sex hormones.

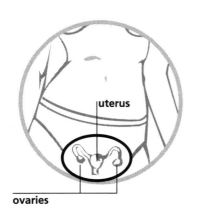

The two primary hormones manufactured by the ovaries are *estrogen* and *progesterone.* Estrogen is actually a family of hormones that perform slightly different functions, but are closely related and are generally referred to collectively simply as estrogen. Estrogen and progesterone work closely together, and are responsible for a number of processes throughout a woman's body, such as the development of female physical characteristics and stimulation of the processes that occur during menstruation. During pregnancy, progesterone helps prevent miscarriage and prepares the mammary glands for the secretion of milk. Estrogen and progesterone play an important part in the maintenance of healthy bones, with the loss of estrogen at the time of menopause being one of the primary contributors to osteoporosis in women.

Other hormones have a more indirect effect on bones, such as those produced by the digestive tract, which aid in the absorption of nutrients, including calcium and vitamin D. While all these hormones play an important role in building and maintaining bone, estrogen — or the lack of it — has perhaps the greatest impact on whether a woman will develop osteoporosis.

From Puberty to Menopause: Estrogen at Work

At the onset of puberty, usually between the ages of 11 and 13 in females, the reproductive organs begin functioning. As the ovaries start producing estrogen and other female sex hormones, obvious physical changes will occur. The young woman will begin menstruation, and the effects of estrogen will soon be evident in the development of what are called *secondary sex characteristics.*

These characteristics include growth of pubic hair and pigmentation of the nipples. As a young woman passes through puberty, she will experience gradual changes in body shape, such as a widening of the hips and enlargement of the breasts. An increased level of estrogen also contributes to changes in the growth plates at the ends of long bones, resulting in the rapid increase in height experienced during the adolescent years.

Of course, one of the primary functions of estrogen is its role in the menstrual cycle and reproductive process. In menstruating women, estrogen levels fluctuate throughout the month. In the first half of a normal 28-day menstrual cycle, while the ovum (egg) is developing in the ovary, the estrogen level increases and stimulates the lining of the uterus (the *endometrium),* causing it to thicken. Around the midpoint of the cycle, estrogen levels drop as *ovulation* occurs: The follicle (sac) containing the ovum ruptures, and the egg is released from the ovary. The now-empty follicle becomes the *corpus luteum,* which secretes another female hormone, progesterone. If the egg is not fertilized and thus pregnancy does not take place, hormone levels fall. The lining of the uterus breaks down and is shed in the discharge referred to as menstruation.

Estrogen and Bones

During the nearly 40 years — from puberty to around age 50 — that a woman's ovaries are producing estrogen, this hormone helps protect her bones. Although the exact mechanism by which estrogen helps slow bone loss is still under study, experts do know that estrogen helps to counteract the bone-destroying effects of the parathyroid hormone. By inhibiting the activity of the parathyroid hormone, estrogen slows the bone resorption process: Less bone is broken down and the overall rate of bone loss is significantly slower.

Researchers have recently found that estrogen may also play a role in the formation of new bone. There is some indication that estrogen may stimulate osteoblasts, because estrogen receptors have been identified in these bone-building cells. Researchers have found that bone cells have receptors for **androgens**, the male sex hormones, as well. The direct effect of hormones on bone-formation cells is still unclear.

As a woman approaches her mid- to late forties she may begin to experience symptoms that indicate a change is taking place in her body. It is usually during these years that the ovaries gradually slow — then nearly halt — the production of estrogen.

The Menopause Years

Before the actual onset of menopause, a woman may notice that her monthly menstrual cycle has become irregular, and she may experience a decrease or increase in her menstrual flow. This period in which the ovaries are slowing production of estrogen, sometimes experienced while a woman is still in her forties, is called **perimenopause**. Perimenopause can last for several years, ending when a woman has her last menstrual period. *Menopause* officially begins when a woman has not experienced a menstrual flow for twelve consecutive months. The average American woman reaches menopause at around age 51.

There are indications that the body is losing its supply of estrogen. While as many as 25 percent of women pass through menopause with little or no trouble at all, others are bothered by chronic and sometimes severe temporary problems that can significantly interfere with their daily lives. The symptoms of menopause are by no means the same in every woman, or for that matter, in every culture. While about 75 percent of American and Canadian women report experiencing hot flashes (sudden intense sensations of heat most commonly felt in the face and upper body), they are so rarely experienced by Japanese women that there is no word in their language to describe it. Researchers attending a National Institutes of Health workshop in early 1993 discussed this cultural phenomenon, citing differences in diet and exercise as a possible explanation.

Some of the most common physical effects of estrogen loss are:

Hot flashes   Most North American women (about 75 percent) experience these sudden sensations of heat in the neck and face during perimenopause, and possibly into the first few years beyond menopause. Hot flashes can last from just a few seconds to a few minutes or longer, and can recur several times a day. The intensity, frequency and duration of hot flashes vary by individual, with some women having only a few hot flashes weekly.

Hot flashes can occur at night, and may awaken a woman to a perspiration-drenched pillow. Some women experience insomnia during this period, finding it difficult to get enough sleep due to the discomfort of these night sweats.

Painful sex   The tissues of the vagina lose moisture and shrink in size. The clitoris and vulva also diminish in size, and intercourse may become painful.

Skin problems   Some women experience a thinning and drying of the skin, while others may experience adult acne or skin that is overly sensitive to touch or pressure.

Urinary tract infections   Shrinking vaginal tissues provide less protection against bacteria, which contributes to an increase in urinary tract infections among menopausal women. These infections are often accompanied by a burning sensation during urination and vaginal itching.

Depression and mood swings   Emotional problems as a symptom of menopause are thought by many experts to be a myth. These experts believe that depression is no more prevalent among menopausal women than other women the same age who have not yet experienced menopause. It is possible that the emotional changes experienced at perimenopause are due, at least in part, to a lack of sleep resulting from night sweats and other symptoms that disrupt a normal sleep pattern. There is also the emotional impact that arises from the woman's feelings of stress and lack of control over the changes occurring in her body. It can be an emotional time, and the experts have yet to agree whether this is attributable to chemical changes or solely due to a combination of physical discomfort and emotional stress.

The duration and severity of the temporary symptoms associated with estrogen deficiency vary from woman to woman. Some women, if they experience discomfort at all, are relieved when it passes within a few weeks or months. Other women have reported menopausal symptoms for as long as five years or more.

Premenopausal Estrogen Deficiency

A small number of women experience an estrogen deficiency — and associated symptoms — even though they are decades away from the expected age of menopause. One reason can be excessive physical exercise that results in a cessation of menstruation, called *amenorrhea.* Other women may experience what is referred to as *premature menopause.* For reasons that have not yet been identified, women in their thirties — and as young as in their twenties — have ovaries that stop working, just as in normal menopause. Researchers speculate that, at least for some of these women, the problem may lie in the immune system: Antibodies may mistake the ovum for foreign material and attack the egg follicle as it would a virus.

If a woman is not certain that she has entered perimenopause, or if she is younger than 45 years old, she can undergo a simple blood test to detect estrogen deficiency. The test measures the level of *follicle-stimulating hormone (FSH)* in the bloodstream, with an elevated level indicating a loss of estrogen.

One of the most serious effects of estrogen deficiency is not physically obvious, but may have the most impact on a woman's life in later years: **Without the protective benefits of estrogen, a woman can lose 2 to 10 percent of her bone mass each year in the first six to eight years of menopause.**

Male Menopause

*W*omen aren't alone in their struggle with decreasing sex hormones at the age of menopause. Recent studies indicate that male behavior and physical condition are also affected by hormones — or a shortage of them. Doctors in England have recently begun treating men for the symptoms of midlife hormone deficiency. The men and their doctors feel that moodiness, lowered sex drive, irritability and fatigue can be alleviated with testosterone therapy.

Just as estrogen is a bone-friendly hormone for women, testosterone helps protect bone in men. While men do not generally go through a period of rapid hormone loss like women experience at menopause, they do slowly produce less testosterone as they age. Bone loss attributed to testosterone deficiency is usually seen in men in their eighties or older. In younger men, low bone mass is most often a result of alcoholism or a dysfunction of the testes.

For a woman who experiences an early menopause — one that begins before age 45 — either naturally or as a result of surgery, accelerated bone loss begins much earlier than normal, further increasing the risk of osteoporosis as she ages.

What can a woman do to protect her healthy bones and avoid osteoporosis? Several options are available, but it is highly likely that one of the first steps you and your doctor will take in planning your strategy against osteoporosis is to discuss estrogen replacement therapy.

The Great Estrogen Debate

Most American women who live beyond the age of 50 or so will be faced with the issue of *estrogen replacement therapy (ERT)*. Whether you are approaching the age of menopause or you are still years from it, you may someday be asked to make an important health decision: Should I undergo estrogen replacement therapy to supply the hormones no longer produced by my ovaries?

For decades, this question has sparked debate among the medical community, women's health advocacy groups, the pharmaceutical companies and women themselves. Almost 50 years ago, doctors first began prescribing "hormone pills," as estrogen supplements are sometimes called. It was not until the '60s, however, that estrogen was widely used to provide relief from the effects of menopause.

The popularity of estrogen replacement therapy suffered in the 1970s. Several studies published in respected medical journals indicated an increased risk of several types of cancer in women taking estrogen, including endometrial or uterine cancer. Researchers continued their work and found that the increased uterine cancer risk may be diminished by cutting back on the estrogen dosage and cycling, or alternating, the estrogen with a synthetic version of another female sex hormone, *progesterone*. The synthetic progesterone is called *progestin*.

This combined estrogen-progestin cycle is sometimes referred to as *hormone replacement therapy (HRT)*. The distinction between HRT and ERT is ignored by many, who use "estrogen replacement therapy" as a generic term. In this book, estrogen replacement therapy is the term most often used, because estrogen is the predominant hormone in both types of therapy, and is of primary concern when discussing the prevention of osteoporosis.

The HRT treatment cycle consists of about three weeks of estrogen followed by about two weeks of progestin. The therapy closely mimics the natural hormone cycle that occurs in menstruating women. This facilitates the shedding of the uterine lining each month, and is believed by some experts to avoid the increased risk of uterine cancer, although this has not been clearly established. Women who have had their uterus removed would not require this combination therapy, since they have no risk of uterine cancer. HRT does have a side effect, however: The addition of progestin can cause a light monthly flow resembling menstruation to resume, even though the woman is not fertile. Some physicians lower the progestin dosage to avoid monthly flow, and to alleviate side effects such as bloating and irritability.

Estrogen Replacement and Your Health

In 1989, women on estrogen replacement therapy got another scare: Several studies conducted in Europe revealed that some forms of estrogen may increase the risk of breast cancer. Some experts believe, however, that the dosage and type of estrogen used for ERT in the United States do not produce the increased risk revealed in those studies. Unfortunately, progestin does not appear to reduce the heightened risk of breast cancer as it does for uterine cancer, and some scientists feel it may actually increase a woman's risk for the disease. There is no conclusive evidence whether the estrogens prescribed in the United States increase the risk of breast cancer, and the issue continues to be controversial.

Popular opinion among the experts is that estrogen is not a *carcinogen*, a substance that *causes* cancer. Instead, it is believed that estrogen may facilitate the growth of existing cancerous cells, or stimulate cells that could be predisposed to becoming cancerous. You should be aware, however, that some physicians do believe estrogen causes cancer. They cite the fact that the incidence of cancer is higher among long-term estrogen users. In fact, women who have been on long-term (five years or more) estrogen replacement therapy appear to be at greatest risk. Studies do not agree whether the increased risk of cancer persists for a significant period of time after estrogen is discontinued.

Despite its drawbacks, estrogen replacement therapy does have a beneficial effect on bone mass, and it relieves the temporary symptoms of menopause. Estrogen may also do your heart good. Studies have indicated that estrogen can increase the level of high density lipoproteins (HDL) in postmenopausal women. This substance is sometimes called the "good cholesterol." A long-term study found that women who took estrogen reduced their chances of dying from cardiovascular disease by 30 to 40 percent. Another study reported by Harvard University showed that women on ERT had about half the incidence of heart attacks when compared to women not taking the drug. Be advised, however, that studies have indicated that progestin negates these benefits to the cardiovascular system. Research concerning the relationship between ERT and heart disease continues, but substantial evidence points to a decrease in heart disease in women on estrogen replacement therapy.

W*omen have a problem sticking with estrogen replacement therapy over the long haul. Experts estimate that even in those countries where it is widely used, only about one in three women who are candidates for the drug use it on a long-term basis.*

Both ERT and HRT have unique benefits and drawbacks. Which — if any — therapy you and your doctor choose must depend on your personal needs and your health history, including your family history of cancer and heart disease.

The Estrogen Replacement Drugs

Several different formulations of estrogen are prescribed in estrogen replacement therapy. The most common ways of taking the hormone are either orally, in tablets, or through the skin using small adhesive patches.

In 1992, the drug most frequently used in estrogen replacement therapy was the most-prescribed drug in the United States. The form of estrogen in that drug is *conjugated equine estrogen*. Simply put, the drug is made up of several substances, some of which are derived from the urine of pregnant horses. The chemicals are joined together in a way that makes them easy for the body to break down. The estrogen tablets range in dosage from .3 milligrams to 2.5 milligrams, intended for daily use. Numerous studies have indicated that .625 milligrams per day is most effective in slowing bone loss, with an increase in dosage not showing any significant increase in benefit to bone mass. Doctors and the drug manufacturers recommend that you take the lowest dose that relieves menopause symptoms and still provides protection against bone loss.

The most commonly used alternative to traditional estrogen tablets are estrogen patches. These contain a form of estrogen called

What's New in Estrogen Therapy

*Y*ou may soon be moving your estrogen supply off the medicine shelf and over with the lotions and creams. An estrogen *gel*, first introduced in France in 1975, has gained such popularity that it now accounts for 65 percent of the French hormone-replacement therapy market. The product, applied to the skin of the shoulders and arms, is currently available in other European countries and may soon be considered for use in the United Kingdom. The manufacturer of the gel, Laboratories Besins-Iscovesco, claims several advantages to using their product:

■ It is significantly lower in cost than other forms of estrogen.

■ It allows the dosage to be adjusted for each individual woman.

■ A majority of women on the product do not experience the monthly menstruation-like flow that is common when progesterone is included in therapy.

Although the drug is currently approved in France only for treating symptoms of menopause, the manufacturer indicates that tests show a reduction in bone loss in postmenopausal women using it. The company may request approval for the drug's use in the prevention of osteoporosis.

estradiol, which is administered *transdermally,* meaning through the skin. The manufacturer recommends placing the patch on any surface of the upper body (including the buttocks or abdomen) except the breasts. The estradiol patches provide estrogen's benefits to the cardiovascular and skeletal systems, with a minimum daily dose of .05 milligrams needed to significantly inhibit bone loss.

Most osteoporosis experts believe that to maximize its positive effects on bone mass, estrogen replacement therapy should begin at the first signs of the onset of menopause, and should be combined with increased calcium intake (about 1500 milligrams of calcium daily). They also indicate that the greatest benefit occurs when estrogen is continued for five years or more, since the greatest amount of bone loss occurs in the first seven years after menopause.

Estrogen Replacement and Bone Loss

How effective is estrogen in slowing bone loss? Studies have indicated that postmenopausal women who have been on estrogen replacement therapy have about half the number of hip fractures as women who have not undergone ERT. Since a hip fracture is a potentially deadly injury, that statistic translates into saved lives. Fractures of the spine and wrist are also significantly reduced by ERT.

Of course, these statistics relate only to a reduction in bone loss and fractures. Experts urge caution and proper medical guidance in all areas of your health, especially when making a decision on estrogen replacement therapy. "Estrogen is currently one of the two FDA-approved treatments for osteoporosis, and appears to be the most effective means of reducing postmenopausal fracture incidence," states C. Conrad Johnston, Jr., M.D., Professor of Medicine and Director of the Division of Endocrinology and Metabolism at Indiana University Medical Center. "However, it has risks, and should be used only by those women who are most likely to benefit. Bone mass measurement should play an important role in making a decision on treatment. The use of estrogen replacement therapy for reasons other than to reduce bone loss is another issue entirely."

As Dr. Johnston mentions, it is recommended that a woman considering estrogen replacement therapy have a bone measurement test to determine her bone density going into menopause. If a woman has low bone density at the onset of menopause, the increased rate of bone loss that can be expected during the first seven years of estrogen deficiency will greatly increase her risk of osteoporosis. While estrogen does not appear to restore lost bone mass, even those women who are well past menopause can benefit from its reduction in further bone loss.

Many physicians and women's health advocates feel strongly that estrogen replacement therapy has been wrongly proclaimed as a fountain of youth that can do everything from making you look younger to keeping you from growing a mustache as estrogen levels decline. The truth of the matter is that menopause — though some of its symptoms may continue for years — is a temporary condition. Unfortunately, one symptom — bone loss — is not temporary. As of today, there are no means of permanently restoring lost bone mass, but estrogen replacement therapy is currently the most effective way of slowing bone loss in postmenopausal women. There is no denying that in the past, when consumers as a whole were more unquestioning, many women received estrogen replacement therapy unnecessarily. By and large, women today are more likely to take the smart approach: Collect the facts, consider the alternatives, weigh the good with the bad and the risks against the benefits. Then, along with expert medical advice from a doctor in whom you have confidence, **make the treatment decision that is right for you as a unique individual with your own needs, lifestyle and medical history.**

The Risks of Estrogen Replacement Therapy

Because estrogen replacement therapy has been used for more than 50 years, scientists have been able to identify many of the problems associated with its use. In addition, some risks and adverse reactions of ERT are extrapolated from data collected on oral contraceptives. This is because the ingredients in birth control pills are similar to the hormones used in ERT.

These are the risks and adverse reactions most commonly associated with estrogen replacement therapy:

Breast and uterine cancer   As discussed earlier, some studies have shown an increase in the incidence of these types of cancer in women on estrogen replacement therapy. The risk of uterine cancer may be decreased by cycling estrogen with progestin. The risk of breast cancer, however, does not appear to decrease with the inclusion of progestin, and it may actually increase the risk of that disease.

Gallbladder disease   Some studies have shown a two- to threefold increase in the risk of gall bladder disease in postmenopausal women taking estrogen.

Liver cancer   Some studies on animals have shown that liver cancer occurs more frequently with long-term estrogen therapy. Conclusive data on people is not yet available.

Thromboembolic disease An increased risk of blood clots has not been proven for users of estrogen replacement therapy. However, there is no doubt that women who take high-dose oral contraceptives containing ingredients similar to those used in estrogen replacement therapy have a significantly increased risk of clots in blood vessels and the heart. These clots can cause a stroke, heart attack or blood clot in the lung, all of which can be fatal.

High blood pressure Oral contraceptives have been shown to elevate blood pressure, and some studies indicate estrogen replacement drugs can have a similar effect.

Contraindications: When Not to Use Estrogen Replacement Therapy

Estrogen can aggravate certain pre-existing diseases and conditions, or produce other negative effects in women who have them. Exercise extreme caution when considering estrogen replacement therapy if you have any of the following conditions:

Pregnancy or breastfeeding Estrogen use by the mother during pregnancy has been shown to increase the risk of congenital defects in the reproductive organs of a fetus of either sex. There is also a risk of future vaginal cancer in female children whose mothers took estrogen while pregnant.

Mothers who are breastfeeding can pass drugs and other substances on to their infants through breast milk, and should therefore avoid any drug therapy unless clearly advised to do so by their physician.

Cancer Women who have some forms of cancer should not consider estrogen replacement therapy unless advised to do so by their physician as part of their cancer treatment.

Some studies have shown increases in the incidence of both breast and uterine cancer in women on ERT, although definitive data has not been presented. Women with breast or uterine cancer in their personal or family medical history are strongly advised against ERT. Estrogen may increase the rate of cancer growth.

Liver disease   Estrogen is metabolized in the liver, and may not be properly processed in persons with liver dysfunction.

Undiagnosed vaginal bleeding   Any woman who has or is currently experiencing vaginal bleeding that cannot be considered normal menstrual flow should not be on ERT, especially if the cause has not been diagnosed.

Heart or blood clotting problems   Women with either of these conditions should begin estrogen replacement therapy only if the specialists treating her for these conditions, in conjunction with her family doctor or gynecologist, have determined that it is safe for her to do so.

Other conditions that may worsen with estrogen replacement therapy   Lupus, migraine headaches, fibroid tumors, metabolic bone disease, fibrocystic disease

Side Effects of Estrogen Replacement Therapy

Some women experience unpleasant, but not life-threatening, side effects when undergoing estrogen replacement therapy. Some of the most common side effects are:

- Nausea and vomiting
- Spotty darkening of facial skin (similar to "mask of pregnancy")
- Bloating and fluid retention, which may aggravate such conditions as asthma, kidney or heart disease, epilepsy and migraine
- Breast tenderness or enlargement
- Increased growth of benign tumors of the uterus
- Depression or moodiness
- Vaginal yeast infections
- Dizziness, faintness and headaches
- Intolerance to contact lenses
- Changes in body weight and sex drive

It is extremely important that any woman considering estrogen replacement therapy receive a thorough physical examination before starting the treatment. Regular breast examinations complemented by monthly self-examination, and yearly gynecological checkups, are strongly recommended. When facing the decision whether to begin estrogen replacement therapy, one of the best investments a woman can make is a visit to her doctor — not for a physical examination, but for an in-depth discussion of the risks and benefits of hormone replacement.

How to Have an Enlightening Talk with Your Doctor

What you have read in this chapter is an overview of the risks and benefits of estrogen replacement therapy. It is very important that you understand both the positive and negative aspects of taking hormones. With that information in mind, have a serious conversation about estrogen replacement therapy with your doctor, and weigh the alternatives. You may be more comfortable with your decision if you schedule a consultation appointment with both your family practice doctor and your gynecologist to discuss the issue.

Expect your doctor to have a strong opinion on estrogen replacement therapy, whether *for* or *against* the treatment. One reason to prepare yourself as thoroughly as possible for your discussion is that, although you want the doctor's input, you must do the decision-making yourself. If you feel strongly one way, but your doctor leans strongly in the other direction, get a second medical opinion. Recognizing this as one of your most important health decisions and educating yourself on the issue are critical to making the choice that is right for you. You and your doctor form an important partnership and, as in any effective relationship, two-way communication is the key to success.

Here, then, are some pointers that may help you get the information you need in order to make this crucial decision, and to help you feel confident that the decision you make is the right one:

■ Read as much as you can about the issue before seeing the doctor.

- Talk to others who have had the treatment that you're considering.

- Contact a women's health center or large hospital in your area for a list of support groups that may have information on menopause, estrogen replacement therapy and osteoporosis.

- Make a list of the points that you want to cover during your visit. Check them off as you get the answers you're looking for, and don't move on to the next point until you fully understand the answer to the question you've just asked.

- Do your homework and be ready to discuss your family medical history as well as your own, especially illnesses such as cancer.

- Schedule an appointment just for your talk. Don't try to cram in your questions at the end of a routine visit — the doctor may want to answer all of your questions, but may be pressed for time with other patients waiting. It's better to have some time set aside just to ask questions and to discuss the issue of estrogen replacement therapy thoroughly.

- Be open-minded and listen to what the professionals have to say, but make up your own mind. You will be living in that body for the rest of your life, and its care and maintenance are up to you.

Other osteoporosis treatments are available. Although none thus far is as effective as estrogen in slowing postmenopausal bone loss, they are good alternatives if you can't take estrogen, or choose not to. No matter how you feel about estrogen replacement therapy, explore the alternatives and know what your options are.

In the next chapter you will learn about other forms of drug therapy used in an osteoporosis treatment program. If you cannot or choose not to participate in estrogen replacement therapy, one of these treatment options may be the partner you need to help slow bone loss after menopause.

CHAPTER 6

Drug Treatments for Osteoporosis

*M*embers of the baby boom generation —
the oldest of whom are approaching the
age of menopause — are once again
reaping the benefits of being a huge
demographic force. The medical research community is responding
to the massive number of Americans who will reach retirement age
during the first 20 years of the new millennium: Based on the 1990
census, the Census Bureau projects that nearly *30 million* women
will be between the ages of 55 and 74 in the year 2010. About
another 22 million will be in their menopause years, ages 45 to 54.
Even though the elderly consume a great deal of our health care
expenditure now, they are the fastest-growing segment of the population. By the year 2000, they will be the major consumer of our
health care dollar. A primary reason for the high cost of caring for
the elderly is the growing epidemic of osteoporosis.

Forces have been put into motion that may soon provide even
more new methods for the prevention, diagnosis and treatment of
osteoporosis. The Women's Health Initiative of the National
Institutes of Health, which got underway in 1993, is but one

example of the new focus being placed on issues affecting the health of women and the elderly. That effort is part of a decade-long study that will involve more than 150,000 women. It focuses on three issues: cardiovascular disease, cancer and osteoporosis. The business sector — pharmaceutical companies and manufacturers of diagnostic machines, for example — are never a group to ignore demographics. They also are hard at work on key health concerns like osteoporosis.

Private and government money earmarked for the study and research of significant health issues is greatly in demand, to say the least, and the competition for these funds is fierce. Only in the previous decade has osteoporosis become a serious contender in the ongoing fight to obtain research funding. The past failure of the scientific communitiy and the government to recognize osteoporosis as a serious public health concern, and to appropriate funding toward its study, is painfully apparent in its limited treatment options. As of 1993, only two drug treatments for slowing bone loss had been approved by the Food and Drug Administration (FDA): *estrogen replacement therapy* and *salmon calcitonin,* a synthetic variation of a naturally occurring thyroid hormone. Even those options are not viable treatments for everyone: Women with a family history of breast cancer, and men suffering from osteoporosis, are not acceptable candidates for estrogen replacement therapy; and calcitonin may produce unpleasant side effects in some patients. Physicians making an aggressive attempt to treat their osteoporotic patients often have to "borrow" drug therapies approved for other bone diseases and to create innovative treatment strategies based on the resources at hand.

Experts agree that a standard of care for the osteoporosis patient hasn't been established yet. There's still too much that is unknown about bone loss, and each doctor treats patients with what he or she has found to be effective. Things are looking up, however. A great deal of research has gotten underway within recent years, which should soon lead to more treatment options for doctors and their patients. Osteoporosis is now a key issue at the National Institutes of Health; there is more focus on women's medical issues and greater willingness to commit health care dollars to women's health.

Learning the Lingo

Bone resorption
The result of the action of the osteoclasts, the cells that break down bone. In a balanced bone-remodeling process, the osteoclasts break down bone, releasing calcium and trace minerals to be resorbed into the bloodstream. The osteoblasts, or bone building cells, respond to the resorption process by building new bone to replace that removed by the osteoclasts.

As the body ages, especially in the years following menopause, the resorption phase goes out of balance with new bone formation, and bone loss occurs. Many of the drugs currently being studied for the treatment of osteoporosis are directed at slowing the resorption process and/or increasing bone formation.

Intervention
Any treatment method used in an attempt to *intervene* in the progress of a disease. An osteoporosis intervention slows the process of bone loss.

There is no magic pill that cures osteoporosis. In this chapter you will learn about methods of slowing bone loss that are currently in use, as well as those that are still under study. Some of these drugs are in the experimental stage, while others are very close to being approved by the Food and Drug Administration for the treatment of osteoporosis. As stressed in previous chapters, the process of halting and even possibly *reversing* bone loss involves a *total treatment program*, with each component complementing the others. The four partners in an osteoporosis treatment program are: **drug therapy, hormone therapy, exercise and diet.**

What Can Drug Therapy Do For Me?

It is *never* too late to start a treatment program that will help you slow or halt the loss of bone mass. Whether you have just recently been diagnosed with low bone density, or have already experienced osteoporotic fractures, there are treatment options open to you. Long-term studies have yet to prove that osteoporosis patients can permanently decrease the risk of fracture by undergoing drug therapy, but substantial data shows that treatment can effectively slow or prevent further loss of bone, allowing patients to hold on to the bone mass they already have.

Some physicians do feel strongly that the right treatment can actually *increase* bone mass, however. "I am currently in the minority, but I believe that osteoporosis is both preventable *and* reversible," says Robert Lang, M.D., Medical Director of the Osteoporosis Diagnostic and Treatment Centers in New Haven and Bridgeport, Connecticut. "In a treatment program that takes into consideration the needs and desires of the patient, I have seen increases in bone mass in women as old as 80." Dr. Lang cautions that such positive results are not universal nor even predictable. "Every patient is different. What works for one person may not produce significant results in another. Treatment for osteoporosis must be *individualized,* with each patient participating in the types of therapy that fit her lifestyle and physical condition."

To arrive at a treatment program that will work best for you, it is important to form a partnership with your doctor. The previous chapter offered some tips on how to have an effective conversation with your doctor, and the same principles apply here. Prepare for a consultation with the doctor as you would for a business meeting:

- Schedule a specific time just to discuss your treatment options.

- Become informed on the subject before your visit.

- Note specific issues that you would like to discuss.

- Be prepared to discuss your personal medical history and that of your family.

- Remember that you are in charge of, and responsible for, your own health care.

According to the American Medical Association's "Patient Bill of Rights," you have the right to respect and dignity, as well as the right to "discuss benefits, risks and costs of appropriate treatment alternatives."

Since most women confront the issue of bone loss around the time of menopause, the first treatment option discussed with you will probably be an increase in calcium intake along with estrogen replacement therapy, which was detailed in Chapter Five. (Most osteoporosis treatment programs include an increased calcium intake — commonly 1,500 milligrams daily from dietary sources and supplements combined.)

For men suffering from osteoporosis, and for women who are unable or unwilling to take estrogen, other treatments are available. The medical community and experts on osteoporosis refer to various treatment options as *interventions*, meaning that they *intervene* in the progress of a disease. A number of different interventions are used by physicians attempting to treat patients with osteoporosis.

"We definitely need more interventions," says C. Conrad Johnston, Jr., M.D., Professor of Medicine and Director, Division of Endocrinology and Metabolism at the Indiana University Medical Center. "Just as in treating an infection, you need as many choices as you can get because no one drug is perfect for everyone."

The first interventions you will learn about in this chapter are those that are currently used by a large number of doctors treating osteoporosis patients in the United States. The last few drugs included are innovative or experimental treatments. The greater the risk of osteoporotic fracture, the more aggressive the intervention. This means patients with advanced osteoporosis are more likely to receive innovative treatment in an effort to prevent further injury.

So, which treatment option is best? It's the one that works best for you. If you or someone you care for has osteoporosis, become as educated as possible about the available options. Don't be afraid to talk to your doctor about the drugs that he or she recommends — an informed consumer wants to know what she's buying and what she's putting into her body.

Prescription Drugs: The Long Road from Laboratory to Medicine Chest

The Food and Drug Administration's approval process for new drugs requires that a manufacturer prove its product is an effective treatment for specific diseases or conditions. Some drugs already in the American marketplace have been shown in studies to be effective for treating osteoporosis, but they are currently approved by the FDA only for the treatment of other diseases. A physician in the United States is given discretionary leeway, however, and may prescribe any FDA-approved drug to any patient for the treatment of any disease or condition.

Obtaining FDA approval — whether for a new drug or for a new use for a drug already on the market — is a lengthy process. Before final approval is granted, clinical trials and other testing have long since been completed, and the treatment has been firmly established as effective. The pharmaceutical company that manufactures the drug, however, cannot market it as being effective for the treatment of any disease except the one for which it has already been approved

Testing New Drugs

*C*linical trials are closely supervised tests that use volunteers to determine the effectiveness and safety of a new drug. The participants undergo innovative treatment that may not be available to the public for months or years.

Volunteers are solicited for clinical trials in a variety of ways, such as magazine and newspaper ads, physician referrals and articles in newsletters apt to be read by the target group. For osteoporosis trials, participants are provided appropriate medical tests and the drug therapy at no charge. They must meet requirements that usually include age, previous treatment history and bone mass below a specific level. The results of these trials are published in medical journals, presented at specialized symposiums and reported by drug manufacturers. Physicians rely on these sources to stay current on the status of innovative osteoporosis treatments.

by the FDA. This prevents the pharmaceutical company from educating physicians about other uses for the drug. Therefore, doctors — and patients — must make a special effort to stay current on optional drug therapies for osteoporosis.

If you and your doctor agree that an alternate drug may help you avoid a debilitating injury, your doctor has a right to prescribe it for you. Before including any drug in your osteoporosis program, ask the doctor to discuss with you the four main concerns of a physician when prescribing a drug to a patient:

- **Efficacy:** Is the treatment effective? Does it work?

- **Cost:** Is this treatment within the financial means of the patient?

- **Compliance:** Will the patient stick with the treatment? Is the treatment inconvenient, uncomfortable or too complicated for the patient?

- **Safety:** Is there potential harm to the patient from this treatment? Does the benefit of treatment outweigh any potential adverse reactions or negative side effects?

Be aware that the information contained in this chapter is for educational purposes only, and is not a recommendation of any drug's effectiveness or safety. Use of drug therapy, whether FDA approved or new and experimental, is a choice that must be made between a patient and her doctor. Generally, the more innovative interventions are used in treating patients with advanced osteoporosis, for whom the possibility of a life-threatening injury is real and immediate.

As with any form of therapy for any disease, the benefits of these treatments should be weighed against the risks of not being treated at all.

How Drugs Work to Fight Osteoporosis

Many of the substances used to treat osteoporosis are *hormones,* produced by a network of glands called the *endocrine system.* The endocrine system regulates such vital body functions as digestion, blood pressure, menstruation, metabolic rate and many others — including bone remodeling.

The focus of much study on osteoporosis treatments has centered around the bone remodeling process — how hormones work to stimulate the osteoclasts, the cells that break down bone, and the osteoblasts, the cells that build new bone. Some interventions for osteoporosis work by repressing the osteoclasts, therefore reducing the amount of bone broken down. This type of intervention is called an ***anti-resorptive agent.*** Since this form of intervention is not believed by most experts to produce permanent increases in bone mass, it should be considered most effective for maintaining *existing* levels of bone mass. In this way, anti-resorptive agents can help avoid initial osteoporotic fractures or help reduce additional injuries in patients who have already had fractures. Patients with a high rate of bone turnover (as determined by the blood and urine tests described in Chapter Four) appear to reap the most benefit from intervention with anti-resorptive agents. Bear in mind, however, that this beneficial effect is not uniform throughout the skeleton. An increase in mass or slowing of bone loss in one skeletal area, such as the spine, is usually not reflected to a corresponding degree in another area such as the hip or forearm.

The bone-destroying phase and the bone-building phase of bone remodeling are normally tightly coupled. The problem with anti-resorptive agents is that the decrease in bone resorption also eventually brings about a decrease in bone formation. Thus the entire remodeling process slows, and the rate of ***bone turnover*** decreases. This decrease could ultimately result in older bone overall, and can prevent the repair of minuscule microfractures, which further weaken bone and contribute to fractures. Once experts know how bone cells communicate and can uncouple the breakdown and building phases of bone, they can successfully target therapy.

Other interventions, including some of the more innovative therapies, are called ***bone formation-stimulating agents.*** These drugs increase both the bone remodeling rate and the activity of the bone-building cells, the osteoblasts. Although all osteoporosis interventions in this category are considered experimental, experts believe that these drugs hold the greatest promise of actually increasing bone mass, rather than just halting bone loss.

A significant challenge in finding an effective bone formation-stimulating agent, however, lies in building new bone that is as strong and fracture-resistant as bone formed *without* drug intervention.

Osteoporosis Drug Therapies

Described here are the drug therapies most commonly used to fight bone loss. Estrogen replacement therapy and calcitonin are the two drugs currently approved by the FDA for treating osteoporosis. Of the remaining drugs listed, some are in the marketplace with FDA approval for the treatment of other diseases; others are still under study and not yet approved by the FDA.

Calcium

Calcium is a key component in *preventing* osteoporosis, with adequate intake of calcium being one of the best things you can do to build peak bone mass in your teens and twenties. Calcium is also a vital partner in any type of osteoporosis therapy. When combined with vitamin D supplements, it is considered by many experts to be the best form of treatment for osteoporosis patients over the age of 75.

Calcium makes up much of the physical composition of bone. Calcium phosphate crystals become embedded in the bone matrix in the **mineralization phase** of bone remodeling. Calcium is also a vital nutrient, carried in the bloodstream, which performs several functions throughout the body. Normal bodily functions cause the loss of calcium: It is excreted in urine, feces and sweat. If lost calcium is not replaced through the diet, the result is a lack of sufficient calcium in the bloodstream. When the body cannot get the calcium it needs from the blood, the parathyroid gland releases hormones that step up the bone resorption process in order to release some of the calcium stored in the skeleton. So calcium works to protect bone in two ways: Adequate calcium intake strengthens bones during the mineralization phase of bone remodeling; and sufficient calcium in the bloodstream slows the bone resorption process.

Studies disagree whether increasing your calcium intake above the normal dietary guidelines, or **recommended daily allowance (RDA)** will increase bone density if you have already reached peak bone mass (at about age 20 or so). Among osteoporosis patients, supplemental calcium is most effective in slowing bone loss in those adults who have low dietary calcium intake and in the elderly.

Treatment with calcium alone has not been proven in clinical trials to reduce fractures, and it does not effectively slow menopausal bone loss due to estrogen deficiency. However, calcium *is* universally recognized as substantially increasing the effectiveness of other osteoporosis interventions.

Calcium is safe, inexpensive and readily available through diet and supplements. Calcium has its drawbacks, however. It may cause stomach and intestinal irritation, including constipation and flatulence. Excess calcium is detrimental to bone: It can decrease the absorption of manganese, a trace metal that is necessary for normal bone, and it may also increase the incidence of kidney stones in patients who are prone to them. A complete look at calcium and how to fight osteoporosis with a healthy diet can be found in Chapter Eight.

Calcitonin

This hormone is found in over a dozen different forms of life, including humans and fish. In humans, calcitonin is produced by the thyroid gland and helps regulate the amount of calcium released from bone into the bloodstream. The form of calcitonin used in treating osteoporosis is called *salmon calcitonin*; not because it is derived from salmon, but rather because it is manufactured to resemble the amino acid structure of calcitonin found in this fish. Salmon calcitonin is about 50 times more potent in slowing bone resorption than the hormone produced by your thyroid.

Calcitonin is an anti-resorptive agent, meaning that it prevents bone loss by suppressing the breakdown of bone by the osteoclasts. When there is a high level of calcium in the bloodstream, the thyroid secretes calcitonin. The hormone works directly on the osteoclasts to decrease their activity. Calcitonin also has been reported to have a pain-relieving effect in patients who have experienced vertebral fractures.

Some studies have indicated an actual *increase* in bone mass in postmenopausal women using calcitonin. Conservative researchers maintain that it is effective only in preventing further bone loss, since any increases in bone mass appear to level off in one to two years. Calcitonin is primarily effective on trabecular bone (the major component of the vertebrae of the spine). Research has not yet shown that salmon calcitonin has a significant effect on the loss of cortical bone. Long-term studies that would determine if calcitonin therapy can decrease the risk of fractures have not been completed.

If you decided to start calcitonin therapy now, you would require several injections each week of the usual suggested dosage, 100 I.U. (international units). Some doctors administer smaller doses, about 50 I.U. given three times per week. This makes calcitonin treatment less expensive, and these physicians believe there is no significant change in effectiveness. Effective calcitonin therapy requires that the patient get at least 1,000 milligrams of calcium each day through diet and supplements.

A number of patients have formed a resistance to salmon calcitonin in long-term therapy, probably because of the effect of antibodies within the immune system. Lowering the calcitonin dosage and using *cyclical therapy* (providing intermittent rest periods in which the drug is not taken) may help reduce the development of resistance.

Treatment with manufactured forms of *human calcitonin* is less likely to invoke a resistance response, though the structure of human calcitonin makes it less potent and therefore less effective in slowing bone loss. Forms of human calcitonin are used to treat other bone disorders such as Paget's disease, a condition that results in the abnormal formation of bone.

Salmon calcitonin can put a dent in your pocketbook — the cost of therapy may exceed $2,000 per year. Some patients taking this drug experience temporary side effects such as nausea, skin rash, frequent urination and flushing of the face and hands, and there is a risk of inflammation at the injection site.

Salmon calcitonin has been approved by the Food and Drug Administration only in injectable form, but studies are underway on a calcitonin nasal spray. (Oral and transdermal — through the skin — forms are also currently under study.) Already available in Europe, the nasal spray appears to have the same bone-saving and pain-relieving benefits provided by the injectable form, and studies indicate that a resistance response to the nasal spray is less likely. The nasal spray is currently in clinical trials; indications are that it will be ready for submission to the FDA approval process in 1993 or 1994. Osteoporosis experts are enthusiastic about the availability of nasal spray calcitonin, hoping that it can fill a gap in treatment options for women who refuse estrogen replacement therapy, and men who suffer from osteoporosis.

Bisphosphonates

Bisphosphonates, also called *diphosphonates*, belong to a class of compounds that are *adsorbed* (attracted and retained) to the calcium phosphate crystals within bone tissue. When the osteoclasts break down the bone crystals coated with bisphosphonates, the compound is released and quickly impairs the osteoclasts' ability to break down bone. Once adsorbed to these crystals, bisphosphonates remain in the skeleton for many years.

While they are not hormones like estrogen or calcitonin, bisphosphonates are anti-resorptive agents. Thus, it was previously accepted that bisphosphonates worked directly on osteoclasts. In early 1993, however, Dr. Herbert Fleisch of the University of Berne, Switzerland, revealed some surprising news at the International Conference on Osteoporosis. Dr. Fleisch reported that bisphosphonates may actually work by blocking signals from the osteoblasts, the bone formation cells. These signals would normally activate the breakdown of bone by the osteoclasts. This news fueled speculation that new drugs could be developed to target osteoblasts. While bisphosphonates inhibit the resorption process, they allow the bone formation stage to continue, resulting in an increase in bone mass. Whether this increase is permanent remains to be proven through the long-term study of patients undergoing bisphosphonate therapy.

As of early 1993, the only oral bisphosphonate available in the United States was *etidronate* (also called *etidronate disodium*), a drug approved by the FDA for the treatment of Paget's disease of the bone. Etidronate has been in use for over a decade, and has shown considerable promise as a treatment for osteoporosis. It appears to be most effective in slowing trabecular bone loss and decreasing spinal fractures.

Patients with advanced osteoporosis appear to reap the greatest benefit from etidronate therapy. In fact, some studies of etidronate as an intervention for osteoporosis have shown increases in spinal bone density of as much as 4 to 5 percent in a two-year period. Etidronate users in one of those tests suffered about half as many vertebral fractures as the group who did not receive the drug. Further studies are needed, however, to determine whether etidronate can have a positive effect on bone mass in the hip and other skeletal sites. The initial research shows significant improvement primarily in areas with a high concentration of trabecular bone, such as the spine.

The positive effects of etidronate on osteoporotic bone loss have been noted in two-year studies. The results of four-year studies will be published in the *New England Journal of Medicine* in late 1993. Ongoing research will reveal whether etidronate can significantly reduce osteoporotic fractures.

Etidronate has a downside — it inhibits the mineralization of newly formed bone if used continuously for an extended period of time. Cyclical therapy with this drug counteracts this effect, slowing bone loss while avoiding the damaging effect on new bone. The etidronate therapy cycle consists of two weeks of etidronate followed by 11 to 13 weeks of calcium supplements. This 13- to 15-week therapy cycle is based on the bone remodeling process: From the start of osteoclastic activity in one microscopic area of bone, to the completion of the mineralization phase in that same tiny area, takes roughly 90 days.

Etidronate is relatively inexpensive, costing less than $50 per month in most areas, and it is taken orally. No serious adverse effects have been noted in the decade that etidronate has been used to treat patients with Paget's disease of the bone, or in clinical trials when used as a treatment for osteoporosis. Bisphosphonates may soon be an effective intervention for men with osteoporosis, and an alternative for women who are unable or unwilling to take estrogen.

Etidronate is not easily absorbed and may irritate the stomach and intestines, causing temporary nausea. To maximize its absorption, foods (especially those high in calcium) must be avoided for about two hours before and after taking the drug, as must vitamins with mineral supplements and antacids that have a high metal content (such as aluminum).

Bisphosphonates remain in bone tissue for years, and the long-term effects, such as toxicity, are unknown. Whether the halting and reversal of bone loss are permanent, and what happens to bone if therapy is discontinued, are also unknown. Experts express concern about possible over-repression of bone remodeling by this drug. This could result in a larger proportion of older bone throughout the skeleton, and the inability of the body to repair minuscule fissures in bone called microfractures.

A great deal of research is centering on bisphosphonates. Etidronate has been used in several European countries as a treatment for osteoporosis, and is in the final approval process by the FDA for that use in the United States. **Second-generation** bisphosphonates are also currently under study. Second-generation drugs have the same basic composition as the original drug but with slight modifications, usually to increase effectiveness, eliminate a side effect or otherwise improve its performance.

High hopes ride on these new drugs — studies indicate that second-generation bisphosphonates may be able to slow the resorption rate even more than etidronate. The first-generation bisphosphonates inhibit bone resorption only slightly more than they slow bone formation. The new drugs appear to improve on that ratio: They cause bone to be resorbed at an even slower pace, while interfering less with new bone formation; the result is a greater net gain in bone mass.This means that dosages can be increased and patients may be able to take the drugs on a continuous basis, rather than intermittent treatment with cyclical therapy.

While the names of these new bisphosphonates are very similar, each is a different drug produced by a different manufacturer: alendronate, residronate (the second-generation etidronate), pamidronate, clodronate and tiludronate. The competition among these drug manufacturers is fierce, with huge financial gain looming in the future. The FDA recently added a twist to the proceedings, however. It altered the requirements for approval of any new osteoporosis drug: The manufacturer now must supply data indicating the drug's effect on *fractures*. Alendronate, in its manufacturer's effort to comply with this new requirement, is currently being evaluated in what is the largest clinical trial ever done on osteoporosis.

Called the FIT (Fracture Intervention Trial), the alendronate study examines the drug's effect on both the prevention and treatment of osteoporotic fractures. The FIT began in 1992, and more than 6,400 postmenopausal women (ranging in age from 55 to 80) will take part in the study before its completion in 1996. During the term of the study, another 25,000 women — while not actively involved in the trial — are being studied to gather information on osteoporosis and other aspects of women's health.

Second-generation bisphosphonates also appear to maintain bone mass in patients who have not yet developed advanced osteoporosis. Women just through menopause, and those who take corticosteroids (a medication that causes bone loss) for diseases like arthritis, show slower bone loss when treated with the new bisphosphonates. Because the new drugs would help maintain bone mass in a much wider range of patients, many osteoporosis experts feel that the second-generation bisphosphonates may soon be one of the best alternatives to estrogen and calcitonin in the treatment of osteoporosis.

Calcitriol

When the skin is exposed to ultraviolet radiation from sunlight, several substances in the body change into *active vitamin D*. Vitamin D, which is actually a hormone, facilitates the absorption of calcium in the digestive system. It also increases the amount of calcium that the kidneys put back into the bloodstream — calcium that would otherwise be excreted in the urine.

Calcitriol is a more active form of vitamin D. It has a more powerful vitamin D effect on calcium, increasing the absorption of calcium and elevating its level in the bloodstream. This in turn "appeases" the parathyroid gland, which hormonally stimulates bone resorption when there is an insufficient level of calcium in the blood. Calcitriol, therefore, acts as an anti-resorptive agent.

Calcitriol has been under study predominantly in Europe. At least two studies indicate that calcitriol can reduce spinal fractures in post-menopausal women. One of these studies indicates that women who are mildly to moderately osteoporotic benefit the most from calcitriol therapy. Some researchers believe that calcitriol may also stimulate the osteoblasts, which increases the formation of new bone.

Most American experts feel calcitriol needs additional testing in the United States, and consider this drug experimental until further clinical trials have been completed. They express concern that there is a very small difference between the dosage of calcitriol that improves bone mass and the dosage that has a negative effect, causing excessive calcium levels in the blood and urine. Also, taking too much vitamin D can be toxic.

While further study of calcitriol is needed, additional research may prove it to be another viable treatment option for osteoporosis.

Thiazide Diuretics

Commonly called "water pills," thiazide diuretics are used in the treatment of high blood pressure and other circulatory problems. Researchers discovered that this medication has an interesting side effect: By increasing the amount of calcium in the bloodstream, it acts as an anti-resorptive agent in treating osteoporosis.

Thiazide directly affects the kidneys, decreasing the amount of calcium lost in urine. This makes the drug an effective treatment for women who have *renal hypercalciuria*, a condition in which the kidneys allow too much calcium to be excreted in the urine.

Thiazide diuretics help slow bone loss by increasing calcium in the bloodstream. This increase in calcium signals the parathyroid gland to slow the release of hormones that stimulate the osteoclasts. The net result is a slowing of the resorption process and a decrease in bone loss.

Unfortunately, this positive effect is temporary. The presence of the additional calcium gradually lowers the level of active vitamin D in the bloodstream. Since active vitamin D is necessary for the absorption of calcium in the digestive tract, the calcium level in the bloodstream gradually declines as well. The lower level of calcium causes the parathyroid hormones to step in again; osteoclasts are stimulated and bone loss resumes.

Although the benefit of thiazide diuretics usually peaks in a period of several months, experts hope that further study will reveal methods of extending the positive effects of this drug.

Anabolic Steroids

This family of drugs has gotten quite a bit of bad press in recent years. Its overuse by professional and amateur athletes has been exposed as a major health risk. A derivative of the male hormone testosterone, anabolic steroids stimulate the body's metabolic process of growth. Testosterone is one of the two main androgens (male sex hormones) that stimulate the growth of muscle and bone in males, and are responsible for the greater body size and strength of men as compared to women.

Athletes use the drugs to increase muscle mass with the aim of improving physical performance. Since anabolic steroids also help maintain bone mass in women, some use of these drugs has been incorporated into treatments to slow bone loss, primarily in older patients with advanced osteoporosis. Anabolic steroids are considered to be anti-resorptive agents because of their protective effect on bone, similar to that of estrogen.

While the drugs do appear to slow bone loss and increase bone mass in women, they have proven to have serious side effects, such as liver damage. Steroids can also contribute to androgenic (male) physical characteristics in women, such as facial hair and a deepening of the voice.

Most doctors feel that the risks of steroids outweigh their potential benefits as a treatment for osteoporosis in women, although the drugs may have some benefit to men with osteoporosis. If anabolic steroids are recommended to treat your osteoporosis, ask your doctor to explain why it would be beneficial to include this form of therapy in your treatment program.

Sodium Fluoride

The same compound found in drinking water and toothpaste, sodium fluoride has emerged as a potent bone formation-stimulating agent in the treatment of osteoporosis. High doses of sodium fluoride (it would take as much as three gallons a day of drinking water to affect bone), when combined with calcium supplements, can significantly stimulate new bone formation and increase trabecular bone mass in the vertebrae.

Sodium fluoride acts directly on osteoblasts, the bone-building cells. Fluoride becomes embedded in the mineral crystals as the osteoblasts form new bone. This treatment has proven to greatly increase trabecular bone density, therefore increasing spinal bone mass.

So why isn't fluoride therapy being hailed as the magic pill for osteoporosis? Unfortunately, it appears that the new bone formed with fluoride treatment is seriously defective. Experts believe that when incorporated into the mineral crystals, fluoride affects the quality and structure of the new bone, resulting in abnormally brittle and fragile bone mass.

In a four-year trial of postmenopausal women, fluoride therapy combined with calcium supplements resulted in a 35 percent increase in trabecular bone density in the spine. The bad news is that cortical bone in the forearm decreased 4 percent during the trial, and there was no decrease in vertebral fractures in the women taking fluoride when compared to the placebo (non-medicated) group. Even worse, there was a significant increase in non-vertebral fractures in the treated women.

Indications are that fluoride therapy promotes the loss of calcium in cortical bone in order to build new trabecular bone. Fluoride can also interfere with the mineralization phase of bone remodeling if adequate calcium intake is not maintained throughout treatment. In addition, many patients taking fluoride experience severe stomach upset and joint pain in the lower extremities.

Combination Drug Therapies

At the 1993 International Conference on Osteoporosis in Hong Kong, B. Lawrence Riggs, M.D., professor of Medical Research at Mayo Medical School and Director of the General Clinical Research Center at the Mayo Clinic in Rochester, Minnesota, addressed his colleagues on the possibility of combining formation-stimulating therapy with anti-resorptive therapy. Dr. Riggs indicated that this combination of drugs would decrease bone turnover while increasing new bone formation, which may decrease the risk of fracture. He stressed, however, that additional studies are needed to confirm his analysis.

Studies are currently underway to determine whether the negative effects of fluoride treatment can be reduced, while retaining the bone-building properties that make it a potential ally in the fight against osteoporosis. The use of lower dosages, other forms of fluoride, different methods of administering it — such as a slow-release capsule — or cyclical therapy may improve results. As it stands now, sodium fluoride is not considered an effective treatment for osteoporosis, even though it has been used in the past and may again be used in the future.

Experimental Drugs

A pressing need exists for new forms of therapy that can effectively treat patients with advanced osteoporosis. While anti-resorptive agents are effective in slowing bone loss and maintaining existing bone mass, progress has been limited in the development of drugs that actually promote healthy new bone formation. Bone formation-stimulating agents — including parathyroid hormone and bone growth factors (described below) — are still in the early stages of investigation.

Studies currently in progress on a group of drugs called *estrogen analogues*, or *anti-estrogens*, may prove them effective in the prevention and treatment of osteoporosis. These drugs appear to offer the positive effects of estrogen on the cardiovascular and skeletal systems, while eliminating the negative effects, such as the possible increased risk of breast and uterine cancer. Asked what forms of treatment we should look for in the future, Dr. Riggs replied, "I think estrogen analogues are a promising form of treatment. The beneficial effects [of estrogen] on bone have been maintained, and yet the side effects have been attenuated. This is a new class of drugs that will come onto the field and play a very prominent role in the next five years."

Bone formation-stimulating agents and estrogen analogues, while still in the experimental stages of development, are terms to remember. In the not-too-distant future, one or more of these drugs may make headlines as the new cutting-edge treatment for osteoporosis.

Parathyroid Hormone

The four tiny parathyroid glands are located in the neck near the thyroid gland. They are responsible for monitoring the level of calcium in the blood. An insufficient level of calcium in the blood triggers the release of parathyroid hormone (PTH), which stimulates the osteoclasts. These cells break down bone through the resorption process, releasing additional calcium into the bloodstream.

The use of parathyroid hormone to maintain bone mass may seem like a contradiction, since its primary function is to make the osteoclasts break down bone. This paradox occurs because the osteoblasts are stimulated to build bone by the activity of the osteoclasts. While the osteoclasts have a relatively short life span, the osteoblasts remain active longer, forming new bone for a significantly longer period of time. Thus the parathyroid hormone is a bone formation-stimulating agent, since bone mass is ultimately increased by stimulating the osteoclasts. Parathyroid hormone also increases the amount of calcium returned to the bloodstream by the kidneys, and steps up the production of vitamin D.

Increases in trabecular bone mass of the vertebrae have been observed in clinical studies of parathyroid hormone. One study indicated, however, that some leveling off of the positive effect occurs after a period of about 12 months. Unfortunately, that same study revealed that cortical bone may pay the price for the improvement in trabecular bone, since cortical mass in the bone of the forearm decreased steadily throughout the study. A newer study, however, reveals that a combination therapy of estrogen and parathyroid hormone may avoid the negative effects of PTH on cortical bone. Further research is needed to determine whether parathyroid hormone therapy can decrease fractures.

Growth Factors

Osteoblasts use several substances to expedite their work in the bone-building phase of the remodeling process. These substances are called *growth factors*, and they show considerable promise in the treatment of osteoporosis.

Growth factors are produced by the body and by the osteoblasts themselves. Both types of growth factor are under study, but the growth factors produced by the osteoblasts, called *local hormones*, are currently generating the greater interest in osteoporosis research.

Dr. Riggs addresses the possible use of growth factors to help treat patients with advanced osteoporosis: "We have a huge population of older people, predominantly women, who already have osteoporosis and have experienced fractures. A number of treatment strategies appear hopeful for this population. Perhaps the most hopeful are the growth factors, provided we can find a way to direct them at the bone cells without affecting the other tissues of the body."

Growth factors are one of the few treatment options that may actually allow patients to regain lost bone mass, indicates Dr. Riggs. "Growth factors are proteins made by bone cells which act on surrounding cells to regulate their function. Use of these natural regulators may be more physiologic [similar to normal, healthy functioning] than use of drugs such as fluoride in stimulating new bone formation."

Tamoxifen

This drug is currently on the market in the United States as a treatment for breast cancer. What can a breast cancer therapy do to slow bone loss? Some researchers believe that the answer may lie in a complicated immune reaction that occurs in women as they experience menopause.

A study performed at the Medical College of Georgia in Augusta, reported in 1992, discovered a strong correlation between an immune-disorder enzyme found in white blood cells and the loss of bone mass. Researchers think that after the ovaries stop producing estrogen at menopause, the tiny message pathways called estrogen receptors on bone cells remain empty. This may initiate a complex immune reaction that results in the loss of bone mass.

Tamoxifen comes into the picture because it binds with estrogen receptors, and may help prevent the immune reaction. A large trial is underway to study the preventive effect of tamoxifen on breast cancer in young women who have a family history of breast cancer.

As part of the Women's Health Initiative at the National Institutes of Health, researchers are also looking for any changes in bone mass in the test group.

Tamoxifen is of particular interest because it can either stimulate or inhibit some of the effects of estrogen, and it appears to inhibit those estrogen receptors that are associated with cancer. The hope is that it may also stimulate those receptors that have a protective effect on bone mass.

Tamoxifen may eventually become a substitute for estrogen replacement therapy in women who are unable to take the hormone due to an elevated risk of breast cancer. The development of this drug could provide women with one more option in finding their own personal solution to the great estrogen debate.

Raloxifene

Another of the new anti-estrogens, raloxifene, also shows promise as a future treatment for osteoporosis. Like tamoxifen, it originally was studied as a treatment for breast cancer. Raloxifene also appears to have the positive effects of estrogen on bone and cholesterol, without some of the negative effects. Anti-estrogens may also decrease the incidence of unpleasant estrogen side effects, like nausea. Raloxifene is currently in the trial phase of development.

This discussion of drug therapies should give you a good idea of the osteoporosis treatments available today and new interventions for the future. Some of these drugs are thought to be highly effective, while others need more study to be of use in treating osteoporosis. This information is not meant to replace proper medical advice and care, and should not supercede any advice or instruction given to you by your doctor. Rather, it is intended to encourage productive conversation between you and your doctor, so that you can become an informed partner in managing your own health care.

CHAPTER 7

Stronger Bodies, Stronger Bones through Physical Activity

You know these people: He works hard all day, so he figures he deserves a little "couch time" every evening after work. She works all day, too — at an outside job or in the home. After she cooks dinner, cleans up the kitchen, does a load of laundry and gets everyone ready for bed at night, she collapses somewhere: sometimes in front of the television on the sofa next to him, sometimes in a warm bath. To his credit, he tries to give her a hand now and then — he takes out the garbage, helps with the kids' baths and generally plays referee in the sibling skirmishes that break out during the evening. As the 11 o'clock news winds down, he nudges her awake and they retire for the night.

"Hey," they'd say. "We do more than *that*." Yes, they do. He plays softball once a week and faithfully shows up at the bowling alley on Thursday nights. She walks around the block a couple of evenings a week, and once a month might get through about half of her workout videotape before one of the kids breaks something or locks the dog in a closet.

107

You *do* recognize these people, don't you? If some variation of this lifestyle *doesn't* come close to describing your daily routine, you're probably one of the fortunate and informed few who have made a conscious effort to break away from the runaway train called "everyday life." Sure, it's tough to turn off the television, put on some serious shoes and do a couple of brisk miles around the neighborhood in 30 minutes or so. But even *tougher* is having our bodies disintegrate in front of our eyes from lack of use and neglect.

There is currently no cure for osteoporosis, but you can prevent it, and physical activity is a key component of osteoporosis prevention. It's never too late to start exercising!

Exercise: A Front-Line Defense Against Osteoporosis

Here it is again — the "E" word. Yes, yet *another* reason to get into those sweat pants: **Exercise has been proven to slow bone loss and help maintain bone mass.** In fact, some researchers and other experts on osteoporosis go so far as to state that exercise can actually *increase* bone mass, although definitive data is still forthcoming on that issue. (Be aware, however, that exercise has not been proven to decrease the incidence of osteoporotic fractures.) One fact remains uncontested: **A sedentary lifestyle increases the rate of bone loss.**

When asked what role he feels exercise plays in the prevention of osteoporosis, B. Lawrence Riggs, M.D., professor of Medical Research at Mayo Medical School and Director of the General Clinical Research Center at the Mayo Clinic in Rochester, Minnesota, answered, "Exercise is very important. I think we have been aware for a long time that increased exercise is good, and we've certainly been aware that people with restricted physical activity, such as quadriplegics and astronauts on prolonged space missions, lose bone." Dr. Riggs says it is no surprise that athletes have more bone mass than the average couch potato. "Recent measurements have indicated that muscle mass and bone mass are directly related. It appears that when you exercise, you have the same effect on bone that you do on muscle. Someone who lives a sedentary life — and that is most Americans — probably has lower bone mass because of lack of exercise."

Does it seem to you that a regular program of physical activity is shaping up to be the miracle cure of the twenty-first century; the "penicillin" of the coming decades? The data is sure stacking up that way: Exercise has been proven to protect against heart disease, to have a positive effect on the immune system, to help prevent certain types of cancer, to improve overall mental condition and, now, to *help save your skeletal system.*

As with almost any preventive measure or treatment program, exercise is not a stand-alone savior when it comes to healthy bones: **Physical activity is simply one key component in any program for the prevention and treatment of osteoporosis.** Its effectiveness does not appear to be restricted to any sex or age group. In individuals already living with osteoporosis a program of appropriate exercise, a healthy diet and treatment with medication may arrest bone loss. Combined with a diet rich in calcium and vitamin D, exercise can effectively reduce bone loss due to aging. In menopausal or post-menopausal women, exercise and a healthy diet complement estrogen replacement therapy, which can greatly reduce bone loss attributable to hormone deficiency.

Everyone can participate in — and benefit from — physical activity. Improvement in bone density has shown up in studies performed on virtually every age group. The U.S. Department of Health and Human Services reported a study of young twins, in which the twin who engaged in an exercise program showed an increase in overall bone mass. In other studies, middle-aged women who took part in specially designed exercise programs showed a significant decrease in the loss of bone density when compared with non-exercising women of the same age. Older women are by no means excluded from the benefits of physical activity — in a study involving a group of osteoporotic women over the age of 69, the effects of exercise on bone mass were gratifying, with *increases* in mass of nearly 4 percent in the targeted bones.

This is merely a sampling of the studies that indicate exercise has a positive effect on bone density. Osteoporosis experts hesitate to

Learning the Lingo

Aerobic   Literally means "with oxygen." Describes any activity that is continuous and rhythmic in nature and elevates the heart rate to within the target zone for at least 20 minutes. Aerobic exercise uses the large muscle groups of the body.

Impact   The force with which the feet hit the ground. Used in describing weight-bearing activities such as running, jogging and aerobic dance.

Intensity   The amount of stress an activity places on the cardio–vascular system.

express a blanket statement that exercise will *add* density to bones. Most will agree, however, that placing demand on the bones through physical activity will help prevent *further* bone loss.

Dr. Riggs comments, "While there is a lack of hard data on the effect of exercise on osteoporosis, one of the few areas of total agreement is that exercise is beneficial. The only disagreement is *how* beneficial."

Exercise pays dividends to your bones in ways that may not be immediately obvious. Here are just a few ways that a regular program of the right kinds of exercise can help protect bone health:

- Building muscle strengthens those layers of softer tissue that help protect your skeletal system from falls and other injury.

- Coordination and balance are improved by exercise, thus reducing the likelihood of a fall and resulting fracture.

- Exercise helps control body weight, allowing exercisers to eat a healthier, more varied diet.

- Emotional stress is reduced. Emotional stress leads to the release of adrenal hormones that break down bone, resulting in a loss of bone mass.

■ As overall fitness improves, the amount of "down time" due to illness decreases. Periods of inactivity such as extended bed rest have been proven to cause a loss of bone mass.

■ Exercise increases the bone remodeling rate, maintaining a "younger" skeleton that includes a greater percentage of newly remodeled bone.

What Is Exercise?

Webster's dictionary has several definitions for the word *exercise*. The one best describing the use of the word in this book is: *"bodily exertion for the sake of developing and maintaining physical fitness."* But physical fitness itself is a broad term. In order to narrow our focus, let's say that the goal of this chapter is to introduce those types of exercise that contribute to *skeletal fitness.*

In some cases you may very well be able to modify your skeletal fitness program to provide other benefits, such as improving your cardiovascular system. After all, the goal of any type of exertion is to achieve maximum reward for your effort. Toward that end, watch for tips throughout this chapter that will maximize the cardiovascular benefits of the exercises you choose for your fitness program — but only if your doctor has indicated that you are physically capable of that level of exertion.

Aerobic exercise

Aerobic exercise is an effective way to maximize cardiovascular benefits. By definition, aerobics is a method of exercise that increases the body's demand for oxygen for a period of at least 20 minutes, performed at a level of *intensity* that raises the heart rate to within a targeted range during the entire period. Joining a gym or buying a workout tape isn't the only way to engage in aerobic exercise; many of the exercises included in this chapter can be performed aerobically. Remember to start your program slowly — especially if you have been physically inactive — *gradually* increasing the intensity of your workouts until you reach 20 minutes of sustained aerobic exercise. Before you begin, learn how to check your heart rate and how to find your target heart rate zone; instructions for both are provided on pages 118-119.

Bearing the goal of skeletal fitness in mind, several types of exercise will be addressed in the following pages. **These exercises have been selected for their ability to place demand, or physical stress, on the skeletal system.**

Exercises for Skeletal Fitness

Weight-bearing exercise

Weight-bearing exercise, according to researchers, is more apt to improve bone mass than any other fitness activity. Weight-bearing simply means that the force of the muscles performing a motion against gravity exerts pressure on the bones, stressing the skeleton. Most weight-bearing exercises are done standing up, since in that position you are *bearing* the *weight* of your body, rather than in a reclined or seated position, in which the weight of your body is borne by the floor or seat. But some calisthenics performed in a seated or reclining position, such as leg lifts, are considered good weight-bearing activities because they use the force of gravity to work against the motion. The weight-bearing exercises most often recommended by exercise experts concerned with the prevention and treatment of osteoporosis include walking, stair-climbing, aerobic routines and jumping rope. Each of those activities will be covered in detail later in this chapter.

Resistance exercise

Resistance exercise is believed by some experts to be highly effective in maximizing or maintaining bone mass. Resistance exercises use an apparatus to make the muscles work harder to accomplish a motion. Whenever you work *against* something in your movement, you're probably doing a resistance exercise. A resistance apparatus can be as simple as a can of peas held in the hand while doing arm exercises, or as complicated as one of the fancy (and scary-looking!) workout machines at the local gym. Other commonly used resistance devices include barbells, dumbbells, elastic or rubber exercise bands and hand or ankle weights. You may see resistance exercises combined with weight-bearing activities, such as hand and ankle weights used in a walking or aerobic dance program. Even the popular stair-climbing machines combine weight-bearing activity with resistance; the apparatus usually allows the user to make adjustments that increase resistance in the climbing action.

Calisthenics

Calisthenics are exercises that use a range of motion to work a targeted muscle and/or bone area. This form of exercise often combines the benefits of weight-bearing and resistance exercise. Calisthenics work by increasing the difficulty of a normal body movement due to a change in position. For example, to bring the head and shoulders forward while standing or sitting is a routine movement, but to lift the head and shoulders from the floor while lying on one's back substantially increases the exertion necessary to complete the motion.

Stretching

Stretching is the simplest and least demanding activity that will be covered in this chapter. It is, however, a very important part of *any* exercise program. Stretching is a method of slow, controlled movement that increases flexibility and range of motion. It is used in the pre-exercise *warm-up* to get the muscles ready for exercise, and again in the post-exercise *cool-down* to help prevent soreness in the muscles. Stretching is also a wonderful way to relax and relieve tension throughout the day.

You will notice that some popular exercises are not mentioned in this chapter. The activities selected are those that appear on nearly every fitness expert's list of exercises judged most beneficial for *skeletal* fitness. Jogging and running, for example, were omitted because of the hazard of bone injury related to those activities.

Some experts believe that *swimming* can help maintain bone mass, while other experts disagree. Nearly everyone agrees, however, that patients who have been diagnosed as osteoporotic, or have already experienced fractures from the effects of osteoporosis, can benefit from exercises that minimize the risk of falling. These patients should also limit the jarring effect, called *impact*, inherent in many weight-bearing activities. Individuals with the limitations described above are encouraged to engage in very low-impact exercises like "water-walking," performed in the shallow end of a swimming pool, or stationary cycling. These types of activities are called *weight-supported* exercises.

Cross-training

Cross-training is of importance to anyone striving to achieve total physical fitness. Cross-training means that you participate in more than one type of activity or exercise. A normal cross-training routine would be to engage in weight-bearing exercise every other day of the week, with resistance exercise and calisthenics done on the alternate days.

Working with people who have been identified as at-risk for osteoporosis, Wendy Kohrt, Ph.D., Exercise Physiologist at Washington University School of Medicine, stresses variety. "Cross-training is probably important. A number of activities can help increase bone mineralization. Of course, each program depends on the physical condition of the individual. A low-impact program would include activities such as the rowing machine and a series of weight-lifting exercises, while someone on a high-impact program would be engaging in stair-climbing, walking or jogging."

Sports

Sports are another wonderful way to stress our bones and reap cardiovascular benefits. Sports that involve low- or moderate-impact weight-bearing activity and have a limited risk of falling are best: Cross-country skiing, tennis, basketball and racquetball are fun ways to get your daily dose of exercise. Be cautious, though — older adults or anyone with low bone density should avoid sports that involve twisting or bending, such as tennis or racquetball.

To summarize, what else can you think of that doesn't cost a lot of money but is good for your heart, your bones and other vital systems, is a great way to keep thin, helps get rid of mental anxiety, stress and depression, can alleviate the symptoms of premenstrual syndrome, may even improve your sex life and makes you feel all-around wonderful? You won't find many things that fill the bill, but exercise can do all that and more.

Whichever of these exercises sounds like fun to you, and whatever it takes to get you motivated about developing a program of regular physical activity: *Get to it!* And remember — even though *some* exercise is better than none, to be truly effective in maintaining a healthy skeleton physical activity must become a habit. Your long-term goal should be to exercise three to six times per week, at least 30 to 60 minutes each time. **The benefits you gain from physical activity end when you stop exercising, so a *commitment* to exercise is essential for a healthy life and strong bones.**

Motivation: The Key to a Successful Fitness Program

First, let's check your overall motivation level. Take, for instance, the most basic of all exercises, one to which we have virtually unlimited access: *walking*. Has it ever occurred to you that we spend the first year or so of our lives trying so hard to learn to walk, then the rest of our lives doing our best not to? Do *you* try every possible alternative before grudgingly giving in and hoofing it somewhere? Take a few moments to answer some questions and we'll see if you qualify for the Unwilling Walker Hall of Fame:

- Do you circle the shopping mall for half an hour looking for the best space in the parking lot in order to avoid walking an extra hundred feet to the store entrance?

- Do you call one of your children from the other room just to get you a soda from the refrigerator?

- Do you find that much of the conversation with your spouse originates from your recliner, and often begins with the phrase, "Hey, hon, while you're in there …?"

- Have you ever, even once, thought about driving the car to the mailbox at the end of your driveway?

- Have you tried to teach the dog to fetch the remote control?

This is a light-hearted look at a serious issue: ***motivation***. Most individuals can *force* themselves to do just about anything once or twice, but in order for exercise to become part of your life you must feel motivated. So far, this book has provided you with some pretty compelling incentives to exercise, but why not sit down right now and make up a *personal* list of reasons?

Today's modern conveniences make it possible to enjoy a lifestyle that is much less physically demanding than in the past. As a result, most of us don't get the minimal exercise we need to stay healthy and fit. Over the years, the need for less physical work has resulted in a more sedentary lifestyle. To keep a healthy balance, we must devote part of our non-working time to physical activity. The good news is that exercise can be *fun*, because a wide variety of activities can give the body the workout it needs.

Your new fitness program should include not just formal exercises, but ways of increasing physical activity in your everyday routine. Look for opportunities to become more active in every aspect of your life.

The Exercise Professionals

No matter what your age or physical condition, there are exercise professionals who can help you tailor a program to fit your needs, your lifestyle, your fitness goals and your physical capabilities. The best way to find one of these experts is to ask your family doctor or the doctor treating you for osteoporosis. In fact, many physical therapists and other exercise specialists require a physician referral. Most hospitals have a physical therapy department, and many of them have an adjunct facility called a ***wellness center*** that can provide excellent guidance in setting up your fitness program.

Several types of health professionals are trained in the science of exercise:

Physical therapist While not a medical doctor, this specialist must be licensed by your state. He or she works closely with orthopedic surgeons and other medical professionals to design and implement a program for returning an injured or disabled patient to maximum physical capability. Some of the tools of a physical therapist's trade are exercise, massage, electrotherapy, ultrasound and hydrotherapy.

Physiatrist This is a medical doctor who specializes in the diagnosis and treatment of muscular and skeletal disorders and diseases. Not to be confused with an orthopedic surgeon, a physiatrist does not perform surgery. Physiatrists are heavily involved in rehabilitation therapy.

Exercise physiologist This degreed professional is educated in the effects of physical activity on the form and function of the human body. Some of these experts have been accredited by the American College of Sports Medicine, which has stringent standards for health and fitness professionals. A goal of the exercise physiologist is to protect the client's good health while assuring an effective exercise program.

An exercise program supervised by one of these professionals is most likely to provide you with a safe, effective workout that is appropriate to your physical condition.

Avoid These Activities If You Have Low Bone Density

Flexion exercises, which involve bending or twisting motions, are not appropriate for individuals who have been diagnosed with low bone density, and should be avoided. They can cause increased compression of the spine and spinal fracture.

Any sport or physical activity that involves twisting or bending should not be part of a fitness program for an individual diagnosed with low bone density or anyone who has had fractures attributable to osteoporosis. Sports like golf, tennis, bowling and racquetball are especially risky for this group of people. Anyone with low bone

How to Find Your Target Heart Rate

*F*eeling your pulse is a simple way that doctors, nurses and *you* can measure the number of times the heart is beating in a specific period of time. When you place your fingers on what is commonly called a **pulse point**, you feel the "thump-thump" of blood pulsing through the arteries, right? *Wrong*. That's a very common misconception — the fact is, you are actually feeling "shock waves" caused by blood being forced from the heart as the heart muscle contracts. These shock waves course along the fibers of the arteries, like vibrations along a tightly strung wire.

The average number of heartbeats per minute in an adult at rest ranges between 60 and 80. The **maximum heart rate**, the level you should not exceed under exertion, can be computed by subtracting your age in years from 220. For example, if Jill is 40 years old her maximum heart rate is 180 (220 - 40 = 180). While exercising, you should strive to maintain your heart rate between 60 and 85 percent of your maximum — this is called the **target heart-rate zone**.

To find your target heart-rate zone, multiply your maximum heart rate by .6 to get the lowest number of beats in your target zone, and again by .85 to get the highest number of beats in your target zone.

Here's Jill's target heart-rate zone:

Maximum heart rate: 220 - 40 = 180

Low rate in target zone: 180 X .6 = 108

High rate in target zone: 180 X .85= 153

Jill should exercise at an intensity that makes her heart beat between 108 and 153 times per minute.

The best way to find and compute your heart rate while exercising is to stop moving and immediately place your index and middle finger *lightly* on the inside of your wrist below the thumb (the **radial artery**, page 119). Count the number of beats felt in 10 seconds, then multiply that number by 6 to figure your **current heart rate**.
You will see individuals who take their pulse at the **carotid artery**

at the side of the neck. This practice is not universally recommended because the finger pressure can cause an inadvertent decrease in blood flow to the brain, resulting in unconsciousness in some people. Other common pulse points are at the inside of the elbow (***brachial artery***) and the back of the knee (***popliteal artery***).

Pulse-taking pointers:

- Take your pulse immediately upon ceasing your activity; it takes only a few seconds for the heart rate to slow.

- Press lightly on the artery to get your pulse; too much pressure will prevent you from feeling the pulse at all.

- Don't use your thumb to check your pulse; it has a strong pulse of its own and may confuse your reading.

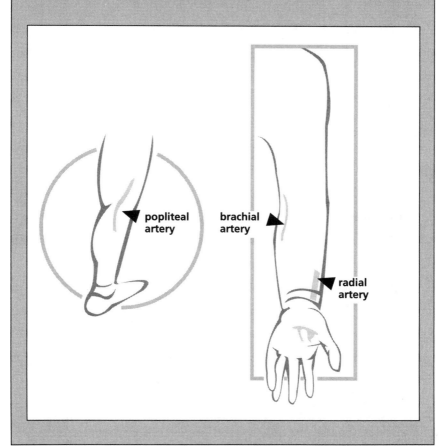

popliteal artery

brachial artery

radial artery

density is strongly urged to exercise under the direction of an exercise physiologist trained to work with people at risk of fracture.

If you plan to exercise without supervision, first become familiar with the warning signs that an activity is too strenuous or taxing:

Signs of Trouble

Sheri Butler, M.A., Exercise Physiologist and Fitness Manager of the Peggy and Philip B. Crosby Wellness Center in Winter Park, Florida, provides this list of warning signs that you may be overdoing it when exercising:

- Nausea
- Light-headedness or dizziness
- Extreme shortness of breath
- Sharp or sudden pain
- Severe muscle soreness that continues longer than three days
- Swelling
- Heart rate that exceeds the maximum in your target zone
- Flushed skin or extreme overheating

Be aware of your body and listen to its signals. If you notice any of these symptoms, stop exercising immediately. Don't hesitate to contact your doctor if any of these warning signs continues for more than five or 10 minutes after you stop exercising. Of course, any severe pain or loss of consciousness require immediate medical attention.

What Type of Exercise Is Best for You?

The answer to that question depends on your age and overall physical condition, as well as the current health of your bones. The types of exercise most beneficial to people in their peak bone mass years, from about ages 15 to 25, will be different from those that are most commonly recommended for an older person, or for someone who has been diagnosed as osteoporotic.

The rest of this chapter discusses in more detail each of the different types of exercise already introduced, and tells which activities are most appropriate and bone-beneficial for each age group. Remember that the most effective fitness programs include various types of exercise: weight-bearing exercise for aerobic and cardiovascular benefits, resistance exercise for intense workouts on specific muscle groups and calisthenics and stretching exercises for increased flexibility and strength.

You've heard this before, but it is a very important point: **Consult your doctor before starting any new exercise program, especially if you have been very inactive, are over 40 years of age, have a heart or vascular condition or are significantly overweight.** Your physical condition is as unique as your fingerprints — the programs and exercises shown here are directed toward those people who have been assured by a physician that they are in good overall health. If you have any reason to suspect that you may have already developed osteoporosis, see your doctor and get tested for this condition *before* starting any exercise program. Those who have been told they have low bone density — *especially* anyone who has experienced a fracture due to osteoporosis — should participate in a fitness program designed and supervised by a licensed exercise professional.

Children

For young, growing bodies to achieve peak bone mass, exercise must begin in childhood. Research studies — or just a glance into the TV room! — indicate that our children are getting too little exercise and not eating enough of the nutritious foods that will allow them to enjoy a healthy body throughout their adult lives. Because the foundation of healthy bones is built during childhood and adolescence, Chapter Nine is devoted to ways you can help your children and grandchildren develop a strong skeletal system. Establishing the importance of fitness and exercise as part of a healthy lifestyle is one of the best gifts you can give to your children.

Adults

The types of exercises most often recommended for an adult in each age group are listed below. If you have been exercising regularly, you already have a good idea of your exercise abilities. If you have been physically inactive, begin slowly and watch out for the signs of trouble listed on page 120.

Adult Phase I (Age 15 to 35)

In these years, your body is building up to its peak bone mass. It is vitally important to do all you can to increase bone density and strength now. There is no second chance — the peak mass attained during these years is what you'll take with you into the period of normal bone loss that will follow.

"Unfortunately, most adults in this age group are extremely weight-conscious, and tend to focus all of their exercise energy on aerobic activities," Sheri Butler comments. "But strength training and other resistance exercises are very important in the overall program."

Low- to moderate-impact weight-bearing activities such as walking, stair climbing, aerobic dance and step-aerobics are recommended at this age. A bone-healthy program should also include some weight training and other resistance exercises. Calisthenics improve muscle tone and stretching exercises are wonderful for improving flexibility. Stretching plays a very important part in the warm-up and cool-down in every workout. The world of exercise is pretty much wide open to individuals in this age group, so select a well-rounded program of activities that will work all of your muscle groups. Don't forget sports: Tennis, volleyball, basketball — all these weight-bearing activities are a terrific way to have fun and get a good workout. Just be sure to proceed at a cautious pace when starting something new.

Adult Phase II (Age 35 to 50)

"Individuals in this age group who are just starting an exercise program should take it slow," recommends Butler. "Include some strength training, and focus on the abdominal exercises, since they help the muscles support the back."

Exercises generally recommended for this age group are the lower-impact activities that do not cause significant risk of falling. Any exercise program should be geared to one's agility and strength. If you have been jogging or playing tennis for years, keep it up unless your doctor — or your body — tell you to stop. If you are new to exercise, walking and stair-climbing are great weight-bearing activities, as are low-impact aerobic dance and step aerobics. Cycling is fine, too. Try to include some *supervised* strength training in your program. While individuals in this age group still consider themselves young, common sense should prevail when new physical activities are introduced. Have your doctor recommend a wellness center or qualified fitness expert who can guide you in setting up your new exercise program, especially if you have been physically inactive.

Adult Phase III (Age 50+ and/or people with low bone density)

"It is very important for individuals in this age group or anyone else diagnosed as having low bone density to make certain that they begin in a *supervised* exercise program," cautions Butler. "We avoid high-impact activities and concentrate on exercises like water-walking to get started."

E*xperts tell us that we are twice as likely to stick with an exercise program if we do it with someone else, so grab a partner and GO!*

Low-impact activities recommended for these adults are walking, cycling and swimming. Most fitness trainers like to see some resistance training for all age groups, so talk to your doctor about activities that are safe for you to include in your program. Stretching exercises to increase mobility are a good idea, as are some calisthenics. Be sure to avoid activities that are hazardous to those with low bone density (page 117).

How Much Exercise Is Enough?

That's a good question and, in regard to skeletal fitness, one that is still a matter of some debate. For cardiovascular benefit, aerobic activity must be sustained for 20 minutes at an intensity that gets the heart pumping within the target heart-rate zone.

Researchers are still evaluating exactly how exercise affects bone. The amount of exercise necessary to stress the bones enough to help maintain bone mass remains unknown. Exercise experts engaged in osteoporosis research feel that the minimum should be 20 minutes per day, three times per week, with optimum benefit gained from exercising 45 to 60 minutes per day, four to five times per week.

Too much exercise is as harmful as not exercising at all. People with low bone density, or those who have not been physically active, should exercise under the supervision of a trained exercise professional.

Athletes who engage in extreme exercise programs, such as marathon training, run the risk of actually losing bone density. This affects mainly women, but also men to a lesser degree. These athletes sometimes develop eating disorders and fail to consume sufficient nutrients to maintain healthy bone. Women are also at risk of amenorrhea, the cessation of menstruation, due to a loss of body fat. When menstruation stops, the bones lose the protective effect of estrogen, and bone loss accelerates.

Exercises of moderate intensity, such as brisk walking, can be sustained by the average person for a longer period of time than a high-intensity activity like aerobic dance or stair-climbing. Set your goals at a level that is within your ability to achieve safely, and watch for the danger signs of over-exertion (page 120).

Another important point from the exercise experts:

Always start your workout with a warm-up and end your workout with a cool-down.

Stretches: Warming Up and Cooling Down

Ah, stretching. Doesn't it feel wonderful, that first full stretch of the morning? Well, it can work wonders throughout the day, too. Stretching is an effective way to alleviate the tension in neck, shoulder and back muscles that accompanies stress. Specially designed stretches prime your muscles for exercise, and help prevent sore muscles after your workout.

For the purpose of warming up and cooling down, perform only *static stretches* — meaning that you stretch to a position, hold it, then release. *Never bounce in the stretched position* — bouncing can strain a muscle. Most exercise experts recommend at least a five-minute stretching routine as a pre-exercise warm-up, and another five minutes as a post-workout cool-down. (A routine consists of all of the following exercises.) A habit of daily stretching will improve flexibility and help maintain a full range of motion in your joints.

STRETCHES: Lower Back and Hips

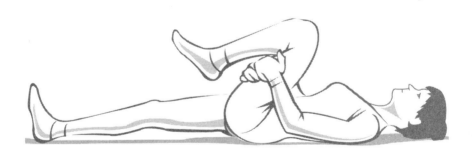

Lie on back. With both hands, grasp the back of one thigh and pull the leg up, knee to chest, with the leg muscles relaxed. The stretch should be felt in the lower back. Hold the position for 10 seconds, then release leg and lower it gently. Stretch the other leg the same way. Repeat seven or eight times, alternating legs.

STRETCHES: Body Stretch

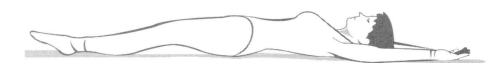

Lie on back. Stretch arms and legs straight out as far as possible. Keep the neck relaxed. Contract abdomen muscles to straighten and flatten back. Hold 10 seconds, relax and repeat five times.

STRETCHES: Back Stretch

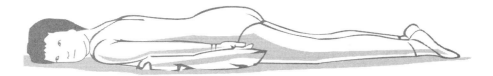

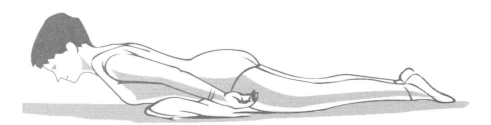

(**NOTE:** This exercise is not for those with low bone density.)
(A) Lie face down, arms at sides, with towel or thin pillow supporting hips and abdomen.

(B) Slowly raise shoulders and head off floor, stretching but not straining the back. Hold three to five seconds. Lower to starting position and repeat eight to 12 times.

STRETCHES: Thighs and Calves

(A) Stand on right foot, with hand on chair or wall for support. Bend knee of left leg, holding ankle with hand and exerting slight pulling pressure. Keep knee in line with the body and opposite leg. The foot should be several inches away from the buttocks. The stretch should be felt down the front of the thigh. Don't bounce the leg, and don't pull so hard that you strain the thigh muscle. Hold for 10 to12 seconds, then release gently. Repeat to stretch other leg.

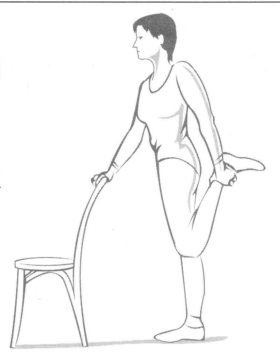

(B) Stand about three feet from wall, bend at hips and place hands against wall. Put right foot back, bending left knee. Keep heel of right foot on the floor and lean forward to feel stretch in right calf and back of ankle. Hold 10 to 12 seconds, then release gently. Repeat to stretch other leg.

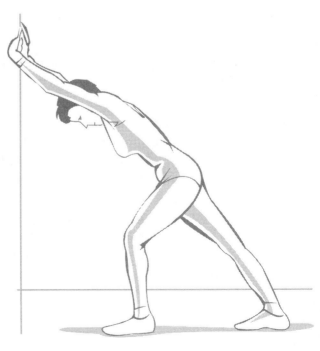

Get Up, Get Out and Move: Weight-Bearing Exercises

This family of activities offers the best all-around exercise, in terms of its positive effects on bone mass and the cardiovascular system. Weight-bearing exercise forces you to work against gravity to exert pressure on your bones, which stresses your skeleton.

Weight-bearing exercises can be varied in intensity, can be done indoors or out, and can be aerobic to boot. But hold on — don't rush out to buy that chartreuse leotard just yet. You don't have to join an expensive health club or buy a videotape to benefit from weight-bearing exercise. You can get that heart pumping and put healthy bone-saving stress on your skeleton with some simple-to-do activities that you can engage in just about anywhere, wearing just about anything.

Weight-bearing exercises require little or no special equipment. Of course, you can have fun using a fancy machine to get that workout, but Mother Nature gave you most of what you'll need to participate in these activities:

- Walking
- Stair climbing
- Jumping rope
- Aerobic programs such as dance or step aerobics
- Stationary cycling

You may notice that we have left out jogging and running, and perhaps some other weight-bearing exercises you were expecting to see on the list. These activities were intentionally omitted because the risks (such as falling or injury to the joints) make them unsuitable for a bone-conscious exerciser. Stationary cycling is included, however. While not performed standing up, cycling offers the benefits of weight-bearing exercise and is frequently recommended by fitness experts for maintaining bone mass.

Well, are you ready to get started? We'll begin with something that you learned to do a long time ago.

Walking: Appropriate for All Age Groups

Serious walkers are almost religious in their devotion. "Before I started walking about a year ago, I was a mess," says Victoria Snyder, a registered nurse for a private-practice surgeon. "Since I started walking a couple of miles a day, *every day*, I feel great. Stress is a thing of the past for me, and I look and feel 10 years younger. If the weather is really terrible and I can't get out for my walk, I *have* to get some sort of workout or I go nuts."

When starting any new exercise program — you'll be hearing this a lot — it is very important to start *slowly*. And even though you may *think* you already know how to walk, don't be too sure — check the illustration on page 132 to assure that you are maintaining good form.

Most experts recommend that a "new walker" begin walking five or 10 minutes a day, four to six times a week; be certain to include a warm-up stretching period before the walk. Then, each week, start adding five more minutes to your daily walk until you're walking between 30 and 45 minutes a day. To get aerobic benefits, work up to a pace that has you walking a mile in about 15 or 20 minutes. Don't forget to do cool-down stretches after walking.

For those who don't feel they have a safe place to walk, or who prefer to work out with a roof overhead, most fitness facilities have treadmills. These machines have a moving surface that allows you to walk in place, and the pace is adjustable to increase the intensity. If

---

The Formula for Keeping FIT

The American College of Sports Medicine offers this handy exercise formula for keeping **FIT**:

F = *Frequency*: 3 to 6 times a week

I = *Intensity*: 60 to 85 percent of your maximum heart rate

T = *Time*: 20 to 60 minutes

So to be **FIT**, exercise for 20 to 60 minutes at least 3 to 6 times per week, at 60 to 85 percent of your maximum heart rate.

Fitness Facts: Walking

- Walking at a rate of 15 minutes per mile burns about 365 calories in an hour.

- A program of walking two miles in 30 minutes, five days per week, burns enough calories to lose about 14 pounds in a year!

- According to the *Guinness Book of World Records*, in 1978 and 1979 Sean Maguire walked from the Yukon River in Alaska to Key West, Florida in 307 days. That's *7,327 miles!*

you prefer to exercise in the comfort of your own home, a treadmill can be purchased at most stores that carry fitness equipment. Try before you buy; the machine should operate smoothly and have readable distance and speed displays.

Your goal for skeletal fitness: Walk 30 to 60 minutes a day, four to six days a week. If you want to achieve maximum aerobic benefit: Walk three miles in 45 minutes, four to six days per week.

To achieve this 15-minute mile, start to step up the pace as you begin to feel comfortable in your program, probably around week six. Try to hold the new pace for a few minutes each day, then *gradually* increase the amount of time at the quicker pace until you've reached your goal.

As you begin to settle into your new walking routine and have reached your goal of three miles in 45 minutes, four or five times each week, you may want to add a dimension of resistance exercise to your walking program by using *hand weights*. Be conservative — a pound or two will do. Simply hold the weights comfortably and swing your arms in a natural rhythmic motion as you walk.

Precautions: Learn how to measure your heart rate (pages 118-119), and check it periodically to make certain you stay in your target range. If you become too winded to carry on a conversation, slow down for a few minutes.

Caring for Your Feet

*W*alter Earnest, D.P.M., a board-certified podiatrist in Orlando, Florida, is a past president of the Central Florida Podiatry Society *and* an avid exerciser. He advises people entering a new walking program to pay attention to their feet: "Before you start walking for fitness, be sure to buy good walking shoes that fit properly." As with any other new pair of shoes, how can you tell whether they will be comfortable in the long haul? "If you can wiggle your toes in your new walking shoes, the heel fits snugly, they don't feel stiff across the ball of your foot and they feel comfortable when worn with thick socks of an absorbent natural material, such as cotton, they are probably a good fit," says Dr. Earnest. "Walking shoes should also be elevated at the heel and curve slightly upward at the toe."

Other precautions to protect your precious feet? "Don't try to grin and bear it if your feet hurt during a walk. Stop and find out what the problem is. Tuck a cotton ball or gauze pad in your pocket until you've broken in your new shoes. If you develop a blister, position the cotton or gauze to protect it from further friction and head home. If the blister pops, apply an antibiotic cream or ointment and cover it with a bandage." Dr. Earnest also recommends periodically checking your feet for deformities such as bunions and corns; seek a foot specialist if these conditions develop.

Here are some other ways to add walking to your day:

- Look for opportunities to walk in place or pace back and forth, like watching television or talking on the telephone.

- Don't take an elevator if you can manage the stairs.

- Don't circle the shopping mall looking for the very closest parking space. If you can park in a well-lit space in a more distant — but safe — area, walk the extra steps to the mall entrance.

Most important of all, *enjoy* your walking program. This is your opportunity each day to smell the roses — so relax, think positive thoughts and *have fun!*

WEIGHT-BEARING: Walking

In Good Form

To get the most out of your walking program, maintain a smooth, even gait. Keep the shoulders aligned with the hips in an erect posture, allowing both the hips and the arms to swing naturally. Bend the arms slightly at the elbow. Try to develop a rolling motion with the foot, landing gently on the heel and rolling through the ball of the foot to the toes. Relax and breathe deeply!

Sample Walking Program

Week 1: 10 Minutes,
4 Times per Week

Week 2: 15 Minutes,
4 Times per Week

Week 3: 20 Minutes,
4 Times Per Week

Week 4: 25 Minutes,
5 Times Per Week

Week 5: 30 Minutes,
5 Times Per Week

Week 6: 35 Minutes,
5 Times Per Week

Week 7: 40 Minutes,
5 Times Per Week

Week 8: 45 Minutes,
5 Times Per Week

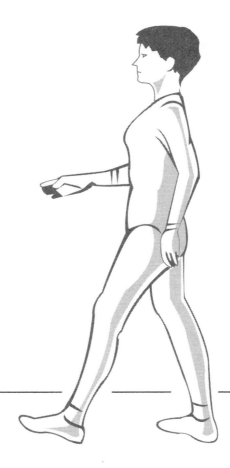

Stair Climbing: Appropriate for Adult Phases I and II

Another healthful activity we've spent our lives trying to bypass! It's a shame, too, because stair climbing is a great weight-bearing exercise that is both low-impact and high-intensity. Stair climbing in the twenty-first century no longer fits the image of football players running up and down the stadium steps. Stair climbing is now high-tech, done on a fitness machine with a control panel that looks, to the exercise novice, like the cockpit of a fighter jet.

Don't be put off by this modern wizardry — stair climbing machines provide a terrific workout that can be adjusted to any fitness level, from beginner to ironman. The pleasant, rhythmic motion of stair climbing is winning over people of all ages. Fitness experts say that time spent on the stair climber is about equal in intensity to time spent running. But stair climbing on a machine has extra benefits:

- It can be done indoors.
- It can be varied in intensity.
- It is a low-impact exercise that's easy on the joints.
- It safely improves balance and coordination, which help prevent falls.

Stair climbing isn't for everyone, though. For exercisers who are significantly overweight, have high blood pressure or suffer knee problems, stair climbing may be too strenuous. People with any of these conditions are strongly urged to check with their doctor before using this equipment.

Everyone who is just starting a program of stair climbing should begin slowly, with the machine on a low or moderate setting. Get instruction from the exercise physiologist at the health facility on the proper use of the stair climber. The action is one of climbing, lifting the legs and pushing down with the balls of the feet. Start stepping no more than five minutes the first time, and add minutes to your workout as you build up your stamina. Experts say that 30 minutes at a moderate setting provide a great workout for the average person, with a five-minute warm-up and a five-minute cool-down each session.

Precautions: Check your heart rate periodically throughout your workout to make sure you stay in your target range (pages 118-119). Don't squeeze the handlebars of the machine tightly; this gripping action can temporarily elevate your blood pressure. Keep an erect posture while stair climbing to avoid placing stress on your back.

Cross-training is a good idea. Stair climbers provide a great lower body workout, but the upper body will need additional activities, such as resistance exercise, to provide a balanced program with maximum benefits.

Jumping Rope: Appropriate for Adult Phases I and II

Jumping rope is another safe, stationary activity that compares to running in its intensity. Jumping rope provides a good aerobic and weight-bearing workout, but is moderately high-impact — it can be hard on the joints if not done correctly. It improves both coordination and balance, and benefits the wrists and forearms.

Other than good shoes (those designed for aerobic dance or cross-training are both good choices), the exerciser will need an appropriate rope. A weighted rope is not recommended. The ideal rope is one of the jointed or beaded variety made of vinyl. These are the easiest to adjust to the correct length, and provide just enough weight to make them easy to handle. To check for proper length, simply stand on the center of the rope and pull the ends upward. Your rope is just right if the ends of the rope reach your armpits.

To reduce impact and intensity when jumping rope, Sheri Butler recommends alternating the feet, sometimes described as "skipping rope." Two-footed jumping increases both impact and intensity. For lower impact, keep your feet within an inch or two of the floor during each jump. Use your wrists and forearms to turn the rope, not your shoulders. Remember, jumping rope is comparable in intensity to running, so work into your jumping program slowly. At first, jump just a minute or two, stopping to take a brief rest of 30 seconds or so before jumping again for another minute or two. Keep moving during your rest period, though — walking in place is a good idea.

When starting out, adjust your jumping speed to a pace that is comfortable. Gradually work up to about two revolutions of the rope per second, or about 120 jumps a minute.

Precautions   Be sure to check your heart rate regularly, especially as a beginner, and adjust your speed up or down to stay within your target heart-rate range.

While you can perform a jumping workout just about anywhere, use a joint-friendly jumping surface. (See Aerobics Programs, below, for specifics.) The area should be free from obstructions that can interfere with the overhead turn of the rope. Practice jumping carefully at first — your feet can become entangled in the rope, resulting in a fall.

Aerobic Programs: Appropriate for Adult Phases I and II

Aerobic programs are as varied as exercise itself. Most fitness clubs, gyms, health spas and even cruise ships offer some kind of aerobics class. Though there are many types and levels, all aerobic programs encompass a structured routine of vigorous movements involving the entire body, and are performed to accompanying music. Some programs incorporate dance-like movements, while others focus more on calisthenics; another type of aerobic program employs a step apparatus to make the body work harder against gravity. Step aerobics is an effective program for beginners (stick with the lower step heights) and provides a great workout.

The key word is *aerobic*, meaning that these activities have been specifically designed to increase the body's demand for oxygen and to provide cardiovascular benefits. To be truly aerobic, the activity must be sustained for a period of 20 minutes or more at an intensity that makes the heart work at a rate within the target heart-rate zone.

Most aerobic programs are broken down into classes that vary in intensity and impact. *Intensity* refers to the level of vigorous activity that takes place in the workout — activity that means reaching and maintaining the target heart rate. *Impact* refers to the amount of jumping and stepping that makes the feet meet the floor with force. In a nutshell, intensity is how hard we work our heart, while impact is how hard our feet hit the floor. For most exercisers, high intensity and low impact make a great combination to look for in an aerobic class — you receive maximum benefit to the cardiovascular system (and work off calories!) while applying limited stress to joints such as the knees and ankles.

When shopping for a new aerobic program you have a number of factors to consider before signing up. Look for programs that have classes for different levels of individual fitness — beginner, intermediate and advanced. The aerobics manager should be able to tell you the levels of intensity and impact for each class, and will help you select the class that best fits your fitness level and goals.

Look for a facility that offers aerobic instructors who have been certified by a nationally accredited organization. To obtain certification, these instructors have successfully completed both a written and a practical examination and are CPR certified. To ask about certified instructors in your area, contact the Aerobic and Fitness Association of America (AFAA), 1-800-445-5950. The American College of Sports Medicine is considered by most in the field of health and fitness as the "gold standard" in the accreditation of exercise professionals. They set stringent guidelines that help ensure a safe, effective workout. To verify accreditation, call 317-637-9200.

You will want the proper footwear for your new aerobic program. Look for a pair of athletic shoes designed for aerobic activity, and use the guidelines on page 131 to get a comfortable fit. Some aerobic exercisers prefer a high-top shoe for added ankle support. To further protect your feet, joints and back, check the floor that you'll be exercising on. Sheri Butler recommends a "forgiving" floor: "Suspended wood or carpeted floors with shock-absorbing material underneath are the best choice. Concrete floors are hard on your body in any aerobic program, and should be avoided."

Most aerobic classes run from 40 to 50 minutes and include a 10-minute warm-up, 20 minutes of aerobic activity and a 10-minute cool-down. Some aerobic classes include an interval of floor exercises or calisthenics. Whatever class you choose, you may wish to add light hand weights to increase intensity as you progress in your program. Ankle weights are not recommended, because they increase the impact level; limit the use of ankle weights to floor exercises.

If you prefer to work out at home, you can invest in an aerobic exercise videotape. If you are just starting your exercise program and are new to aerobics, it is a good idea to get a feel for the proper way to perform the movements and dance steps from a certified instructor. Save your videotape program for later, when you'll have some aerobics experience under your belt.

Precautions   As in any exercise program of significant intensity, participants must learn to keep an eye on their heart rate. If your heart rate during the class doesn't reach the low number in your target heart-rate zone, you need to increase intensity. If your heart rate exceeds the high number in your target heart-rate zone, slow things down a bit. A good instructor will teach the class to monitor their heart rates periodically throughout the workout.

Watch the impact level of the classes you participate in — high-impact activities increase the risk of injury, especially for beginners.

Stationary Cycling: Appropriate for All Age Groups

Like stair climbing, cycling has gone high-tech. While there's certainly a great deal of pleasure in hopping on your bike and taking a leisurely ride around the neighborhood, the workout that can be had from a stationary cycle is almost awe-inspiring. It is easier to get a controlled aerobic workout on a stationary cycle, and it is considerably safer than dodging traffic and avoiding snarling neighborhood dogs. Stationary cycles also reduce the risk of falling for those with low bone density.

WEIGHT-BEARING: Stationary Cycling

In Good Form

To get the most from your stationary cycling workout, maintain an erect posture to avoid strain on your back. Adjust the seat so that it is level and your knee is slightly bent on the full extension of the downstroke.

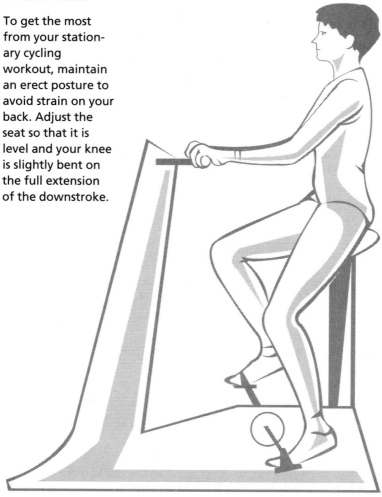

At your local fitness center or health club you may be confronted with a stationary bike that resembles transport of the future. Like a stair climbing machine, it may have a control panel that would look right at home in a fighter jet. These gauges and digital displays provide you with valuable information about your workout: the speed (rpm, or *revolutions per minute*) that you pedal, the level of resistance at which you're pedaling, the amount of time you've been cycling in the session and the number of calories burned during this workout. Have the instructor guide you through your first few sessions on the cycling machine, and help you increase your workout as you progress.

Some machines have built-in cycling routines that automatically vary the level of resistance during your program, intermittently increasing the pedaling force you must use in order to simulate cycling over hills. You select a difficulty level, and the cycle guides you over a varied course. At the beginning and end of the program you will usually experience lighter resistance levels, with the middle of the program devoted to increased resistance.

Some fitness centers, especially those that offer physical therapy, will feature two types of stationary cycle: the standard type with the user sitting in an upright position, and a *recumbent* cycle that allows the user to assume a semi-reclined position, with the legs extended parallel to the floor. The recumbent cycle is popular for older exercisers since it is closer to the ground and therefore easier to get off and on, and the seat provides support for the back.

Beginning cyclists should take it easy, starting with a workout of about five or 10 minutes at a low resistance level. Work up to maintaining about 40 rpm during your session, making sure to check your heart rate early in the workout. Three to four sessions a week will provide you with a great lower body workout that includes aerobic benefits.

As you progress, add minutes to the time you spend on the cycle and gradually nudge up the resistance level. If your cycle doesn't have a program that automatically varies the resistance level, start and end your workout with lower resistance, sandwiching the higher level of resistance in the middle of the session. Cyclists will benefit most from a warm-up and a cool-down of at least two or three minutes, with the period of higher resistance in the middle of the workout gradually getting longer. A good goal for experienced stationary cyclists is a 30 to 40 minute workout, three times per week. As you become more accustomed to your cycling program, you can increase the speed at which you are pedaling to about 60 to 70 rpm.

Should you decide to invest in your own stationary cycle, look for a good solid machine that feels stable. Some stationary cycles feature handlebars that move back and forth, adding an upper body workout. Your new cycle should be comfortable, have non-slip pedals and include gauges indicating speed (or rpm), time elapsed and distance covered. The seat and handlebars should be fully adjustable, and you should be able to select different resistance levels. Be forewarned: The electronic cycles like the ones used by most health clubs and fitness centers are *expensive*, but you can get a similar workout on a much simpler machine.

Precautions   Cycling can be an intense workout, so keep an eye on that heart rate. It is a good idea for beginners to check their heart rate after a minute or so on the cycle, and periodically throughout the workout. Avoid gripping the handlebars too tightly, since that action can temporarily increase your blood pressure.

If you choose to do your cycling outdoors on a "real" bicycle, be sure to wear clothing that will not get caught in the wheels or pedals, and *invest in a good cycling helmet*. A three-wheel cycle, or "adult tricycle," provides added stability for those who are not confident that they can safely handle a two-wheel bicycle.

And remember to cross-train, using resistance exercises or calisthenics, because your upper body doesn't receive a full workout from cycling.

Resistance Exercises

Sometimes called *strength training*, resistance exercise employs an apparatus that makes the muscles work harder to complete a movement. The apparatus may be barbells or free weights, or other equipment as diverse as weight machines, large rubber bands (like a strip of bicycle inner tube) or just a can of soup held in each hand. **Resistance exercises are appropriate for all age groups, as well as for people with low bone density (under supervision).**

Resistance exercise is highly effective in maintaining bone mass. Participants can target particular muscles and, therefore, specific areas of bone. Parts of the skeleton that are at particular risk for fracture as bone loses mass, such as the spine, hips and wrists, can benefit greatly from a program of resistance exercises. Researchers have noted in numerous studies that bone density can be improved with this type of exercise. The results are not restricted to the young and strong. Older patients, including postmenopausal women and nursing home patients, have shown increases in both strength and bone density as a result of programs using resistance exercise.

Inexperienced exercisers who would like to begin a resistance program should learn the ropes from a fitness professional. These activities must be done correctly in order to reap the full benefits of the exercises and also to avoid injury.

Starting your resistance program means taking it easy at first. Fitness experts recommend that beginners start with very light weight, or even no weight at all. Gradually, as you gain strength, you

Fitness Fact: Resistance Training

 n a study performed on elite athletes, researchers found that weight lifters had the greatest bone density of all the athletes tested, while swimmers had the least.

can add more weight to your exercises so that you continue to increase the benefits to bone and muscle. The group of exercises in this chapter will provide you with a well-rounded resistance program for both the upper and lower body.

Resistance exercise has a language of its own: Each time you perform a movement is called a *repetition*, or *rep*, and each series of eight to 12 repetitions is called a *set*. Start your program with three sets of eight repetitions of each exercise, with a rest between each set of about two to three minutes. (Translation: Do an exercise eight times, rest for two to three minutes, do another eight of the exercise, rest for two to three minutes, then do your last eight of the exercise.) Be sure to complete all three sets of each exercise before moving on to your next exercise. If you're using the right amount of weight, the last couple of repetitions should be tough, but possible to do. If you can't complete all three sets or all eight of the repetitions, you may need to cut back on the amount of weight you're using. Your resistance program should be performed three times per week, on alternating days.

The resistance exercises in this chapter require a minimum of equipment, so once you get some expert instruction you will easily be able to follow the program at home. Personal instruction is always a good idea, to make sure you're performing the exercises correctly. Even if you want to exercise at home, a lesson or two at a fitness center will promote maximum benefit and help prevent injury.

Your trainer will teach you to take your joints through their proper range of motion. Move slowly on the way up *and* the way down — don't let momentum carry the movement up, and don't let gravity do your work on the way down. Avoid jerky movements, and don't rush — the slower these exercises are done, the better.

Should you want a more intense workout that can greatly increase the benefit to your skeleton as well as your physique, check out the weight machines at your local health club or wellness center. These include the Nautilus and Universal mechanical machines, as well as the newer electronic machines. They provide excellent resistance exercise targeted to specific areas of the body, and you'll benefit from

Cross Training

A well-rounded exercise program should include all four types of exercise included here: weight-bearing, resistance, calisthenics and stretches. Experts suggest that weight-bearing activity be done every other day, complete with warm-up and cool-down stretches. Resistance training, calisthenics and stretches should be done on the alternate days. Don't overwhelm yourself — work slowly into a program that fits your physical condition, interests and schedule.

the instructor's guidance. Remember, a good health club or fitness center will *always* ask whether you have any special physical limitations, and will review your fitness goals with you in order to design an appropriate program to fit your needs.

The equipment you'll need to do the resistance exercises that follow include an exercise mat, a set of dumbbells or hand weights (one to three pounds each will be fine to start with), and an elastic or rubber exercise band. All of these items should be available at your local sporting-goods or athletic-supply store.

Precautions   Target heart-rate zone and pulse rate are not usually a concern in resistance exercise and strength training, because they are not aerobic activities. Listen to your body, however, and be alert to the signs of trouble described previously in this chapter. And *keep breathing!* Many times you'll catch yourself holding your breath on exertion. Fight that urge and breathe as normally as possible during all the exercises.

Rest between sets. Gripping the weights can temporarily elevate blood pressure, and your muscles will need the break.

Resistance exercises are excellent for building muscle and for stressing the skeleton to maintain bone mass. But for a well-rounded exercise program, you'll need to cross-train with weight-bearing exercise.

RESISTANCE: Dumbbell Raises — Shoulder (Trapezius)

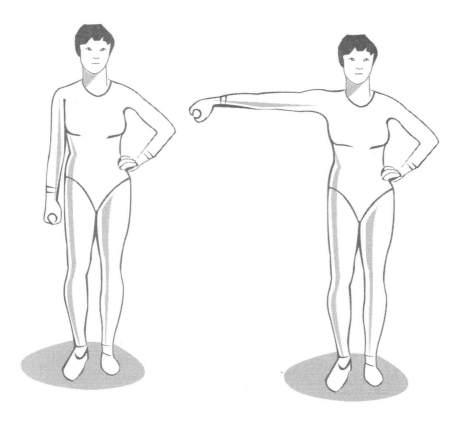

(A) Hold the dumbbell at your side, palm facing inward and arm fully extended.

(B) Lift your arm straight up from your side and away from your body. Lift only to shoulder level — lifting higher can injure the shoulder joint. At this position, your palm should be facing the floor with the elbow slightly bent. Slowly lower arm to starting position. When all three sets are completed, repeat with the other arm.

RESISTANCE: Dumbbell Raises — Back of the Upper Arm (Triceps)

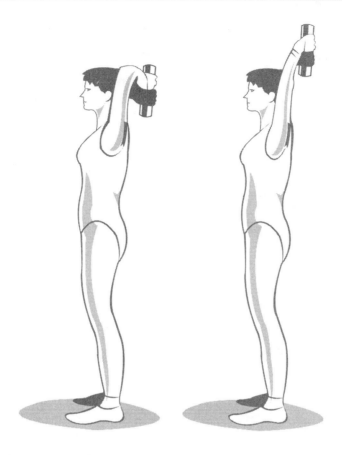

(A) Hold the dumbbell behind your head with both hands, the upper arms straight up beside your head.

(B) Slowly extend your forearms upward, bending at the elbow while the upper arms remain close to the sides of your head. Slowly lower arms to starting position.

Complete three sets.

RESISTANCE: Curls — Front of the Upper Arm (Biceps) and Forearm (Forearm flexor)

Biceps curl

(A) Hold a dumbbell in each hand, with palms facing up at about waist level and elbows at sides.

(B) Slowly raise the dumbbells, then slowly lower them to starting position. Keep elbows close to the waist; do not move them forward.

Complete all three sets before moving on to

Forearm curl

(C) Hold dumbbells as shown for biceps curl, but with palms facing down. Keep the wrists straight. Slowly raise the dumbbells, then slowly lower them to starting position as described in steps A and B.

Complete three sets.

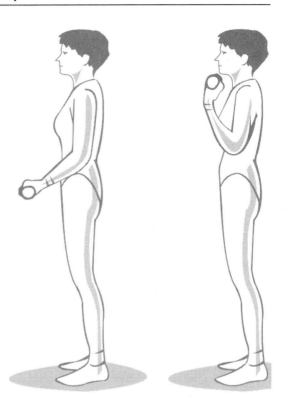

Hand positions

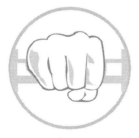

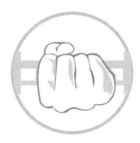

forearm curl   biceps curl

RESISTANCE: Front of Thigh (Quadriceps)

(A) Sit upright in a hard chair, back relaxed but straight, feet on floor, band around legs at ankles.

(B) Lift left leg straight out, extending the foot until the leg is parallel to the floor, keeping other foot on the floor. Slowly lower leg to starting position.

Complete three sets, then repeat with right leg.

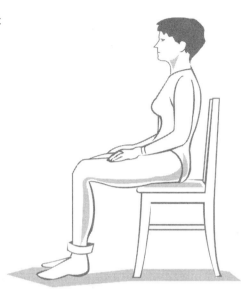

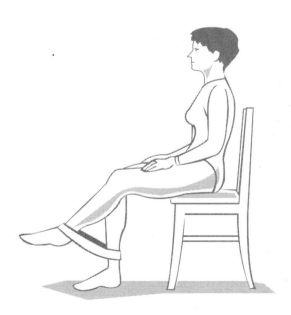

RESISTANCE: Hip and Outer Thigh (Hip abductors)

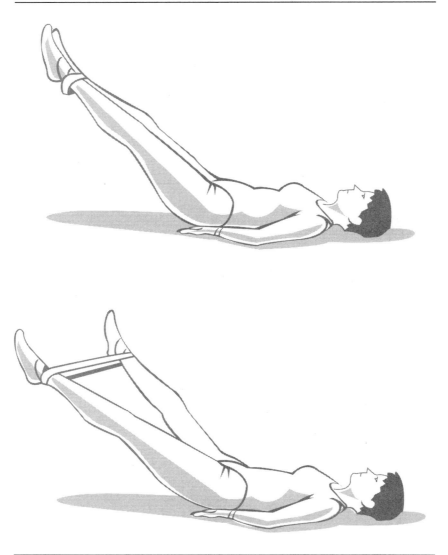

(A) Lie on back. Put band around both legs at ankles. Tuck hands, palms down, under buttocks to protect lower back from overextension. Raise legs off floor several inches, with knees slightly bent.

(B) Move legs apart slowly as far as you can, keeping them parallel with knees slightly bent. Bring legs slowly back together to starting position.

Complete three sets.

RESISTANCE: Hip and Outer Thigh (Hip abductors)

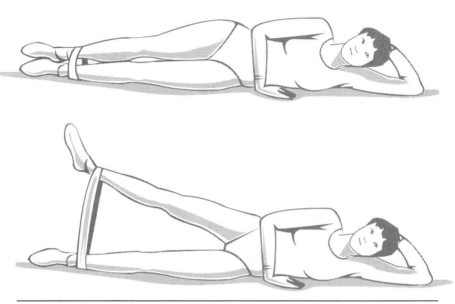

(A) Lie on left side, head propped up with hand. Place the other hand on the floor at about waist level for balance. Place right leg on top of left, with band around both legs at ankles.

(B) Lift right leg as far as you can, with knee facing forward (not up) and foot flexed (not pointed). Slowly lower leg back to starting position. If you find your body leaning forward, bend bottom knee to add stability.

Complete three sets, then turn over and repeat with left leg.

Calisthenics

Calisthenics, sometimes called *floor exercises*, were selected for this book because they can be used to target very specific muscle groups. For example, leg lifts help support the spine by strengthening the abdominal muscles.

Stretches should be done as a warm-up to calisthenics. If you have not been physically active, start by doing just a couple repetitions of each exercise — but do them all. Work your way up to about 20 to 25 minutes of stretches and floor exercises, done three to four times per week.

Precautions   Don't overdo calisthenics; take these exercises at your own pace. Don't bounce; a slow, controlled movement is your goal.

As with any physical activity, if you feel sudden or sharp pain, **stop**. If the pain persists, it would be wise to speak with your doctor.

CALISTHENICS: Chair push-ups — Chest and Back of Upper Arms

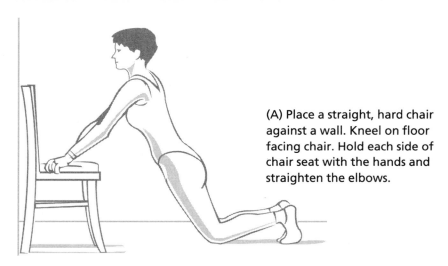

(A) Place a straight, hard chair against a wall. Kneel on floor facing chair. Hold each side of chair seat with the hands and straighten the elbows.

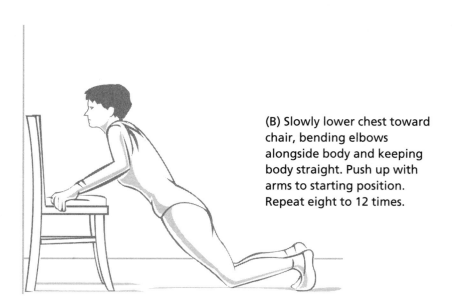

(B) Slowly lower chest toward chair, bending elbows alongside body and keeping body straight. Push up with arms to starting position. Repeat eight to 12 times.

CALISTHENICS: Leg Lifts

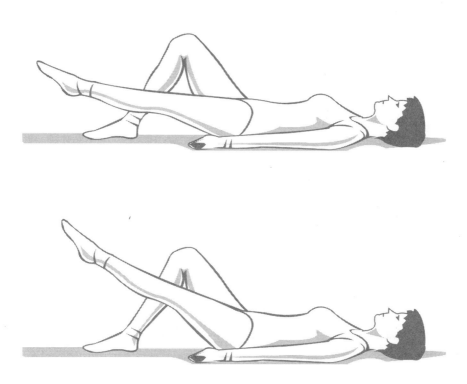

(A) Lie on back, arms at sides. Bend right leg at knee with foot flat on floor. Keep left leg straight with toe pointed, about 6 inches above floor.

(B) Lift left leg up to 18 inches off floor and hold for two to three seconds. Slowly lower leg to starting position. Perform eight to 12 times, then repeat with right leg.

CALISTHENICS: Knee Lifts

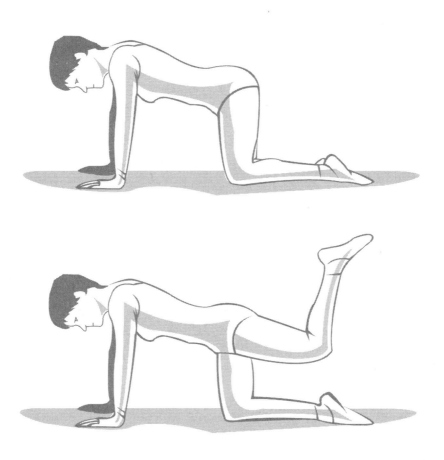

(A) Kneel on floor on hands and knees. Relax shoulders and head, but don't sway or arch back.

(B) Lift left knee straight back, as if pushing at ceiling with foot. Keep knee at a 90-degree angle. Slowly return knee to floor. Perform eight to12 times, then repeat with right knee.

CHAPTER 8

Fighting Osteoporosis with a Bone-Healthy Diet

*A*mericans are obsessed with food. It has long surpassed its unsung status as just a source of energy and nourishment to sustain life. Food has become a passion; we celebrate it with fairs and festivals, use celebrities and sports stars to sell it, and have special organizations to help us manage our love for it. Is it because we so dearly love our food that we often fail to use it to our advantage?

In all aspects of your life you are faced with making choices — and that includes what you eat. That old saying "You are what you eat" holds a deep basic truth about the human body. The dietary choices you make affect every aspect of your physical being, and much of your emotional self. Good health, beautiful skin, shiny hair, a well-proportioned body — all are directly influenced by the food you choose to eat. This is true of healthy bones as well.

Relax — in this chapter you will *not* be lectured about your diet. Most adults know their dietary downfall — whether it be sweets, salty snacks or French pastries — and seldom need others to point it out. What you *will* learn is how to make good dietary choices that

Learning the Lingo

Calorie is a unit of measurement of the amount of energy a food can make available to the body. Fats provide 9 calories per gram, while proteins and carbohydrates provide 4 calories per gram.

Recommended Dietary Allowances (RDA) are the amounts of essential nutrients needed to meet the needs of a healthy person on a daily basis, established by the National Academy of Sciences' Food and Nutrition Board. The table of requirements for each of these nutrients is divided into sex and age categories.

United States Recommended Daily Allowances (U.S. RDA) are the maximum amounts recommended for each nutrient in any of the categories (sex or age). These standards are set by the Food and Drug Administration based on the recommendations of the committee described above. They are the standards listed most often on the labels of packaged foods.

will help you build and maintain healthy bones. First will come a basic lesson in nutrition, then you will move on to information about calcium, vitamin D and other nutrients vital to your skeletal well-being. You will receive pointers on the best ways to supplement your diet if you aren't getting enough of the right kinds of food, and discover which foods steal away vital nutrients. You will learn to spot misleading nutrition labels on prepared foods, and how good — or bad — your favorite foods are in the categories of calories, fat, sodium and calcium.

Learning to use food as a partner in your fight against osteoporosis is a smart move at any age. In order to make truly informed dietary choices, however, you must first understand some of the basic concepts about food and its effects on your body and your health.

Food Fundamentals

Children usually take a health class in elementary school that teaches them about nutrition and the basic food groups. For most adults, that class is the extent of their formal training about food. In fact, a great many people know more about their washing machine than they do about the food they eat.

As an American, you are constantly bombarded with information about food by television, newspapers and magazines. Most of this information is presented courtesy of the manufacturers of prepared foods, who obviously have much to gain by getting you to think that their products are safer, healthier and cheaper than the competitors' products. While the law and consumer protection groups seldom allow food manufacturers to get away with out-and-out lies, advertising agencies working for these huge food corporations know how to stretch and manipulate the truth. For the majority of adults, this means that what we *think* we are eating and what we *really* are eating may be two very different things. Throughout this chapter, you will see examples of how the nutritional value or other aspects of a food product can be masked behind technical terms, misleading labeling and slight misrepresentation of facts.

Regardless of how or why you buy the products that you do, your body needs to consume certain nutrients in order to survive. In most cases, you obtain these vital nutrients from the food you eat. **Foods fall into three major classifications:** *protein, fat and carbohydrate.*

Protein: The Body's Building Material

Protein is used to grow, repair and maintain healthy tissue in the human body. In Chapter Two, you learned that protein forms the basis for new bones. It does that and much, much more — protein is necessary to sustain life.

There are different types of protein, all made up of combinations of 22 *amino acids.* The body cells that manufacture protein can synthesize some of these amino acids, while others, called *essential amino acids,* cannot be created by the body and must come from the food you eat. Foods that provide all nine of the essential amino acids in the necessary proportions are sources of *complete protein.*

Animal products provide most of us with our complete proteins: Meat, chicken, fish, eggs and dairy products are all good dietary sources of essential amino acids. Some plants contain protein, but most lack one or more amino acids or do not have them in the needed proportions. If you are a vegetarian, it is important to educate yourself about food combinations that will supply all of the essential amino acids.

Be aware that protein from animal products has been under scrutiny for its negative effects on health. While hard scientific evidence has not yet been produced, several studies have shown a link between animal products and diseases like cancer and heart disease. One large study conducted by Cornell University looked at the diet of thousands of Chinese as compared to the diet of their American counterparts. In the United States, the percentage of dietary protein intake from animal sources is seven to 10 times higher than that of the Chinese, who get 90 percent or more of their protein from plant products, such as legumes. The heart disease death rate among American men is about 17 times higher than that of Chinese men of the same age. Further studies are needed to determine whether this is partly attributable to high meat intake in the American diet.

The National Academy of Sciences' Food and Nutrition Board recommends that adult males include 63 grams of protein in their daily diet; adult females should include 50 grams of protein daily.

The bones may also suffer from excessive meat consumption. Meat is acidic, and the body pulls minerals — including calcium — from the bloodstream in order to balance the acidity. When the blood calcium levels drop, the body breaks down bone to replace it. Thus, too much meat in combination with too little calcium in the diet can set the stage for bone loss.

No one is advocating that Americans completely stop eating meat;

however, the U.S. Department of Agriculture, in its Food Guide Pyramid released in 1992, recommends that adults limit their intake of meat, poultry, fish, dry beans, eggs and nuts to two to three servings per day, 2.5 to 3 ounces per serving. The Food Guide Pyramid and the major food groups are discussed later in this chapter.

Fat: Do You Really Know What You're Eating?

Fat is perceived as a food ingredient that contributes little to overall good health and has a long list of negative consequences. The truth of the matter is, some forms of fat are essential to sustaining life. There are actually several types of fat, which you may hear referred to by their scientific term, *lipids*. Different kinds of fat perform vital functions throughout the body. Fat comprises a large part of cell membranes and nerve linings. Stored fat provides insulation against heat loss and protects bones and organs. Some bone-friendly hormones, such as estrogen, testosterone and vitamin D, are manufactured by the body from certain kinds of lipids. Dietary fat provides taste and texture to much of your food and is an important source of energy.

Fats are actually made up of a combination of compounds called *fatty acids*, which are made primarily of carbon, hydrogen and oxygen molecules. Dietary fat takes two different forms: Oils, which are liquid at room temperature, and fats, which are solid. All fats and oils contain both *saturated* and *unsaturated* fatty acids. These terms have become very familiar to health-conscious American consumers. Food manufacturers often throw them about, and it is important to learn the differences between the two types of fat.

The terms *saturated* and *unsaturated* refer to the way the carbon atoms are bonded together to make up a fatty acid. When the carbon atoms are bonded together one-on-one, they can attach to the greatest number of hydrogen atoms. Thus they are *saturated* with hydrogen. When the carbon atoms are chained with double bonds, the fatty acid cannot take on as many hydrogen atoms, so it is *unsaturated* with hydrogen. Let's take a look at why this distinction becomes important when making your dietary choices:

Saturated Fats These fats are described as *stable* fats, since the single carbon bonds within their structure make them the most non-reactive of all types of fats. This stability makes saturated fatty acids more difficult for the body to break down and convert into other usable substances. It also makes them more resistant to spoilage; they do not easily become rancid.

The fats in meat, milk, cheese, lard and other animal products contain mostly saturated fats. What surprises many people is that some *plant oils* are made of saturated fatty acids as well. These are called the *tropical oils*: coconut oil, palm oil and palm kernel oil. Tropical oils are heavily used in manufacturing processed foods, although they are not as prevalent today as in the past.

Saturated fats have been labeled as "bad guys" in the American diet. High intake of these fats has been associated in studies with increased cholesterol levels in the blood. Many experts now believe there is a direct relationship between diets high in saturated fats and illnesses such as heart disease and cancer of the colon and breast.

Unsaturated Fats   Because of one or more double bonds in their chain of carbon atoms, unsaturated fats are more easily broken down by the body, and are referred to as *unstable* fats. Usually, the more unsaturated a fat, the softer it is at room temperature; unsaturated fats are primarily the vegetable oils. There are two types of unsaturated fats:

■ **Monounsaturated**: A fatty acid that has only one double bond in the carbon chain is called *monounsaturated*. Oils that contain a large percentage of monounsaturated fatty acids, such as olive oil and canola oil, have received favorable press in recent years. Studies have indicated that substituting monounsaturated fats for saturated fats in the diet may help lower blood cholesterol levels.

■ **Polyunsaturated**: Two or more double carbon bonds make a fatty acid *polyunsaturated*. The more double bonds a fat has, the more unsaturated it is. Corn oil, safflower oil and soybean oil contain mostly polyunsaturated fatty acids. These oils may help lower blood cholesterol levels when used instead of saturated fats in the diet.

All dietary oils and fats are made up of numerous fatty acids, both saturated and unsaturated. The product is classified by the predominant kind of fat: A vegetable oil considered to be polyunsaturated may actually contain as much as 20 to 25 percent

Fat: How much is good?

*T*he Committee on Diet and Health of the National Academy of Sciences' Food and Nutrition Board recommends that no more than 30 percent of daily caloric intake come from fats, with 10 percent or less provided by saturated fats. For an average female who consumes about 2,000 calories per day, no more than 660 calories should come from fats. This means fat should be limited to 73 grams or less per day.

The average male should limit his daily fat intake to 97 grams or less, with a total fat intake of 870 calories.

monounsaturated and saturated fats.

With all the concern over dietary fats, how are food manufacturers handling the pressure? Some continue to use highly saturated palm and coconut oils because they have a long shelf life and easily go through the rigors of processing. While these plant oils *are* cholesterol free — as the product label is sure to proclaim — they are also saturated fats. Why don't manufacturers substitute one of the polyunsaturated oils? Because corn, safflower and soybean oil — the most common polyun-saturates — are difficult to work with in the manufacturing process, and quickly become rancid when exposed to oxygen.

What food manufacturers have come up with is a little technolog-ical hocus-pocus: a process called *hydrogenation*. To make polyunsaturated oils hardy enough to withstand the demands of processing, the double carbon bonds of these fats are broken down and saturated with hydrogen. If not all of the double carbon bonds are broken, the product is *partially hydrogenated*. Hydrogenation stabilizes the oil, making it into a solid fat that is easier to work with, but it also has the unfortunate effect of turning polyunsatu-rated fats into saturated fats. The result: The food manufacturer gets to espouse a product as containing polyunsaturated fats and being cholesterol-free, while you buy and consume a product containing a hydrogenated polyunsaturated fat that is, in reality, highly saturated.

Cholesterol is a form of fat, and as a special dietary concern is discussed in detail later in this chapter.

Carbohydrates: Easy Energy

Carbohydrates are provided by the foods that most Americans consider "the good stuff:" sugars, starchy foods and fruits. Experts estimate that up to 60 percent of the average American's diet consists of carbohydrates. These foods provide the primary source of energy for the body. Carbohydrates are divided into two categories:

Simple carbohydrates   This is the sugar group: table sugar (sucrose), milk (lactose) and fruits (fructose) are some of the dietary sources of simple carbohydrates. Your body expends little effort in converting these foods into blood sugar, or *glucose.* Tissues throughout the body, such as the muscles and brain, use glucose for energy.

Simple carbohydrates are not necessary to produce glucose, however — when pressed, the body can synthesize blood sugar from protein or fat, as well. In fact, a diet that is consistently high in simple sugars can result in such undesirable conditions as obesity and high blood pressure.

When you eat a hot fudge sundae, for example, the body quickly converts the sugars in the food to glucose. The blood sugar level rises and the pancreas responds by secreting *insulin,* the hormone responsible for keeping the blood sugar level within the optimum range. If the body does not need all of the glucose for energy, insulin converts the excess glucose into fat.

> The National Academy of Sciences' Food and Nutrition Board recommends that adults get 55 percent of their daily caloric intake from carbohydrates.

Complex carbohydrates   Primarily *starches* and *fiber,* these carbohydrates are made up of chains of many sugar molecules. Pasta, grains, breads and vegetables contain complex carbohydrates.

It takes longer for the body to digest these foods and convert them into blood glucose. The blood sugar level rises gradually, which helps avoid rapid increases of insulin in the bloodstream. Without the peaks and valleys in blood sugar level associated with simple carbohydrates, foods rich in starches and fiber can help you feel satisfied longer — allowing you to avoid unhealthy snacks between meals that can add fat and calories without providing the nutrients your body needs.

Simple carbohydrates (sugars) are easy-access energy foods for the body, and a diet that is chronically high in these foods can prevent the use of stored fat. One gram of carbohydrate provides about 4 calories. While a candy bar may satisfy your hunger for a short period of time, it lacks the bulk that will keep a growling stomach at bay until your next meal. In addition, the chronic rapid elevation of insulin level caused by excessive sugar intake can result in obesity. Obesity may contribute to the body's forming a resistance to insulin, resulting in an increase in the risk of certain types of diabetes.

Some of the complex carbohydrates, like grains, pasta and vegetables, have considerable bulk, making them great sources of fiber. Fiber, along with cholesterol and sodium, is of special concern to many Americans. Let's take a look at those hot dietary topics.

The Good, the Bad and the Misunderstood

Cholesterol

A soft, waxy substance that is a member of the lipid family, this fat plays key roles throughout the body. It is one of the components of nerve linings, and is the substance from which some bone-friendly hormones are formed — estrogen, testosterone and vitamin D, for example.

Cholesterol comes from two sources: In the average person, up to half the cholesterol in the bloodstream comes from the diet; the rest is provided by a metabolic process in the liver. Therefore, your blood cholesterol levels are dependent on several factors, chiefly the amount and kinds of fat that you eat, the amount of high-cholesterol foods in your diet, lifestyle factors like smoking, and genetics — that is, how much cholesterol your body naturally manufactures.

Cholesterol is carried throughout the body by *lipoproteins*, a combination of lipids and proteins that bind with cholesterol. There are two types of lipoproteins you should be concerned with:

■ *Low-density lipoproteins (LDL)* are the "bad guys," since the cholesterol carried by these lipoproteins is more apt to adhere to the walls of arteries, which contributes to heart disease.

■ *High-density lipoproteins (HDL)* are the "good guys," because they actually help remove cholesterol from body tissues, then pass it on to the liver where it is processed and finally sent into the digestive tract to be eliminated.

The best way for a normal, healthy person to control blood cholesterol levels is to limit the amount of saturated fats in the diet, substituting monounsaturated and polyunsaturated fats like olive, corn, safflower and soybean oil. While some dairy products are high in saturated fat, they are excellent sources of calcium. To lower your cholesterol intake, switch to skim milk products and low-fat yogurt and cheese.

T*he National Academy of Sciences' Food and Nutrition Board recommends that adults limit their cholesterol intake to less than 300 milligrams per day.*

Sodium

Sodium is a mineral that is essential to the healthy functioning of the body: It helps maintain the proper balance of body fluids. Salt cannot be synthesized by the body and therefore must come from the diet. This is not usually a problem, since most foods contain sodium. Other than in your salt shaker, sodium is found in significant amounts in most snack foods, baking soda and baking powder, monosodium glutamate (MSG), canned goods and delicatessen-style meats (like bologna, salami and corned beef).

Excess sodium in the diet can cause fluid retention, which may result in high blood pressure in people with kidney dysfunction. It has also been associated in studies with increased bone loss. In one study, patients on low-sodium diets reduced the level of a biomarker in the urine that indicates bone destruction. Postmenopausal women are especially vulnerable to the effects of salt, since their bodies are less efficient at absorbing and metabolizing calcium and vitamin D. Although the correlation between salt and bone loss needs further study, osteoporosis experts feel that reducing salt may help slow bone loss by increasing the reabsorption of calcium normally lost through the kidneys.

To cut down on sodium, eat fresh and frozen vegetables instead of canned, replace deli-style sandwich meats with their low-sodium counterparts and limit your consumption of foods like ham, smoked meats and fish, pickled foods and salty snacks.

T*he National Academy of Sciences' Food and Nutrition Board recommends that healthy adults consume between 500 milligrams and 2,400 milligrams of sodium per day.*

Fiber

A real boon to breakfast cereal manufacturers, the health benefits of *fiber* — actually a form of carbohydrate — made big news in the late 1980s. Found in a variety of plant substances, from apple pulp and citrus rind to wood chips and vegetable gums, fiber is divided into two types:

■ *Soluble fiber* is fiber that breaks down in water, forming a gel-like substance. It has been reported to have several dietary benefits. Soluble fiber slows the absorption of carbohydrates, helping to moderate the blood sugar level. By binding with bile acids in the intestines, it can decrease cholesterol in the bloodstream, which may lower your risk for heart disease. Studies have also indicated that soluble fiber can decrease the level of bad lipoproteins (LDLs) and increase the level of good lipoproteins (HDLs), which also decreases the risk of heart disease.

Soluble fiber can easily be included in the diet by eating foods like oatmeal. Several soluble fiber products, which are usually mixed with water, are available over the counter. As with other aspects of your diet, it is preferable to get fiber from the foods you eat rather than relying on supplements.

■ *Insoluble fiber*, since it is not soluble in water, does not change as it passes through the digestive tract. It is most valued as a means of adding bulk to the stool, speeding up the elimination of digested foods and increasing bowel movement frequency, and it may help prevent colon cancer. Insoluble fiber is found primarily in the bran layer of cereal grains, such as those in whole-wheat foods.

A kind of insoluble fiber called *cellulose* is extracted from wood. Food manufacturers sometimes add it to bread and other bakery products. Since cellulose has no calories or carbohydrates, it can be used in combination with flour to add fiber and bulk, and it effectively reduces the caloric count of foods by as much as one-third.

Those who want to increase their dietary fiber should do so slowly. Too much, too soon can cause painful gas and possibly nausea. Eat fruits and vegetables instead of drinking juices, eat brown rice instead of white, and switch to whole-grain breads and bakery products. Remember, though: **Excess fiber intake (more than 30 grams per day) can speed up digestion to the point that vital nutrients like calcium are not properly absorbed, increasing the rate of bone loss.**

Last but certainly not least among the food fundamentals are vitamins and minerals, several of which play key roles in the formation and maintenance of healthy bones.

Vitamins and Minerals

Vitamins

Vitamins are organic chemical compounds the body requires for healthy functioning. These micronutrients — nutrients necessary in tiny quantities — are needed for nearly every imaginable process in a healthy growing body, from the healing of wounds to the formation of blood cells. They help convert food into the very fabric of your physical self: Your skin, blood, nerves, organs and bones are all formed and maintained with the interaction of vitamins. While large doses of specific vitamins are not a guarantee of optimum health, a deficiency of vitamins can result in disease and poor health.

Vitamins cannot be manufactured within the body, and thus must be supplied by the diet. Some vitamins, such as vitamins A and D, are oil or fat soluble; others, such as vitamin C and most of the vitamin B complex, are water soluble. Solubility plays an important role in where and how a vitamin is metabolized and absorbed.

Vitamin D, considered both a steroid hormone and a vitamin, is one of the key components in building healthy bone. It helps increase intestinal absorption of calcium from the diet, and helps the reabsorption of calcium in the kidneys. Vitamin D is present in the body in both active and inactive states. Ultraviolet radiation from sunlight activates an inactive form of vitamin D in the skin. While vitamin D is stored in the liver in this partially activated state, it is the kidneys that convert vitamin D into its fully active form.

Vitamin D occurs naturally in fish, eggs and liver, and is added to most milk. Few Americans need vitamin D supplements, because the RDA of 400 I.U. can be met with a well-balanced diet. One cup of milk provides about 25 percent of the RDA for adults. Those who think they may need to take vitamin D supplements should check with their doctor first, since excess amounts of this chemical can be toxic, and may actually *increase* bone loss.

Minerals

Minerals are different from vitamins; they are inorganic substances that exist naturally in the earth. More than a dozen minerals are essential to life and health, with nearly twice that many forming the total mineral composition of the body. Minerals are generally needed in larger quantities than vitamins, and must come from dietary sources. Some of the vital minerals for which an RDA has been established are iron, magnesium, zinc, iodine, phosphorus and calcium.

Some minerals are classified as *electrolytes*, substances that are responsible for maintaining fluid balances and proper functioning of body cells. The primary electrolytes are sodium, potassium and chloride. A number of elements, such as chromium, are not currently classified as essential but are used by the body in small amounts. These are referred to as *trace elements.*

Far from being a trace element, the mineral having the greatest impact on the bones is calcium.

Calcium — the Bone-Building Mineral

Calcium is the most abundant mineral in the body. As you have read throughout this book, calcium is essential for the growth, health and maintenance of the human body. It is needed for proper clotting of the blood, normal functioning of muscles and nerves, and to maintain the heartbeat. At least one study has indicated that a diet high in calcium (1,250 milligrams each day) may decrease the risk of colon cancer.

While your body cannot manufacture calcium, it *does* store it. About 99 percent of the body's calcium is stored in the skeleton. Calcium provides strength and density to the bones, and the loss of calcium is what brings about the weakening of the skeleton that can lead to osteoporosis. When there is not enough calcium in the bloodstream to adequately perform the body's vital functions, the body's calcium regulators kick in.

In response to low blood-calcium levels, the parathyroid glands release a hormone that stimulates the osteoclasts to break down bone. The osteoclasts create tiny cavities in bone tissue, releasing the calcium stored within the bone. The calcium is reabsorbed into the bloodstream, where it is available for use in the vital functions described above. This process of destroying bone to release the stored calcium is called *resorption.*

The osteoblasts move into the microscopic areas of bone that have been excavated by the osteoclasts. As bone-formation cells, they lay down the first form of new bone growth, a matrix made up of a type of protein called collagen. Shortly, calcium and phosphorus from the bloodstream will be deposited into the collagen matrix. Within a few weeks, the calcium and phosphorus will harden into crystals. This entire calcification phase of new bone is called *miner-alization*, and is the process by which calcium is stored within the skeleton. This calcium will be released during future resorption initiated by the parathyroid hormones — and the cycle continues.

What's the best way to hang on to the calcium in your bones?

- Eat a well-balanced diet that includes a variety of calcium-rich foods.

- Get a few minutes of sunshine every day, to help maintain your body's supply of vitamin D.

- Avoid the "calcium robbers" — those foods, drinks and lifestyle factors that can steal away your valuable calcium.

Let's take a look at the stages in our lives when we can best use dietary calcium to help prevent osteoporosis:

Calcium Intake for Each of Life's Phases

Adolescence   During the first few years following puberty, the body experiences a period of rapid growth due to the effect of sex hormones on bones. Experts say that nearly three-quarters of our peak bone mass — the most bone we'll ever have — is built during this period. From adolescence to about age 30, a diet rich in calcium can help build up the skeletal calcium stores. The more bone mass you bring out of this period, the better your defenses against osteoporosis in later years.

The RDA of calcium for adolescents (ages 11 to 24) is currently 1,200 milligrams, with some experts holding the belief that young adults in these bone-building years should increase their intake to 1,500 milligrams to maximize bone density. (See Calcium Supplements, page 175.)

Premenopause   From about age 30 until menopause, bone loss in women occurs at a rate of about 1 percent per year. (Men usually hold this low rate throughout their lives, which is why they are at less risk for osteoporosis.) While the current RDA of calcium is 800 milligrams for adults, the National Institutes of Health and the National Osteoporosis Foundation agree that the adult RDA should be increased to 1,000 milligrams per day. Of course, special circumstances (like early menopause or bone-robbing diseases and medications) may warrant additional calcium intake. The RDA for pregnant or lactating women is 1,200 milligrams per day.

Menopause   In many ways, menopause is a unique period in a woman's life. She is dealing with a number of chemical changes in her body, not the least of which is the loss of the protective effect of estrogen on bone. The first five to seven years after menopause are particularly hazardous to her skeleton, since most of the loss of bone mass due to estrogen deficiency will occur during this period.

While the need for adequate calcium in the diet continues throughout a woman's life, there is a conflict of opinion among osteoporosis experts concerning calcium's role in estrogen-deficiency bone loss. Some studies have indicated that supplemental calcium can help slow the loss of bone during this period, while others have come up with results clearly to the contrary. Nearly all agree, however, that estrogen replacement therapy, not calcium, is the first line of defense against osteoporosis in the years immediately following menopause. (See Chapter Five for an in-depth look at menopause and estrogen replacement therapy.)

The most commonly recommended daily calcium intake for post-menopausal women who are on estrogen replacement therapy is

Recommended Daily Calcium Intake

Life Stage	Age	RDA* Milligrams Per Day
Children	Birth - 6 months	400
	6 - 12 months	600
	1 - 10 years	800
Adolescents and Young Adults	11 - 24 years	1,200
Adults	25 + years	800**
Pregnant and Lactating Women	All Ages	1,200

*Recommended Dietary Allowance, National Academy of Sciences' Food and Nutrition Board, 1989.

A consensus of The National Osteoporosis Foundation and National Institutes of Health recommends **1,000 milligrams daily for adults age 25 and over, and 1,500 milligrams daily for postmenopausal women not on estrogen replacement therapy.

1,000 to 1,200 milligrams. The National Institutes of Health and the National Osteoporosis Foundation recommend that women not on estrogen replacement therapy increase their intake to 1,500 milligrams per day.

The Senior Years The elderly have special conditions that increase their need for calcium. As a group, they tend not to eat as much as other adults; some are impoverished and their diets suffer as a result. Others live alone and simply don't bother to eat. The body's ability to maintain healthy bones decreases with age due to a combination of factors:

■ The intestines become less efficient at absorbing vital nutrients.

■ Parathyroid activity may increase, which stimulates the bone-destroying cells.

■ The elderly take more medications that may interfere with the absorption of calcium.

■ The body becomes less efficient in the absorption and activation of vitamin D.

■ The elderly are more likely to need extended periods of bed rest, which can drastically increase the rate of bone loss.

A common practice among doctors treating elderly osteoporosis patients is to include vitamin D supplements (usually at least 400 I.U. daily) along with 1,000 milligrams or more of calcium.

No matter what your age, it is always preferable to get your RDA of calcium from dietary sources rather than relying simply on supplements. Your calcium-rich foods will also contain other nutrients needed for a healthy body, and a well-rounded diet is a significant part of any osteoporosis prevention or treatment program.

Calcium and the Food Groups

Many of us were taught in school about the "Four Basic Food Groups," and our mothers followed these guidelines in planning the family meals. Well, how Americans think about food and nutrition has changed considerably in recent years. To keep pace with this transformation, the United States government recently changed its recommendations for a healthy diet. The four basic food groups are no longer our national guidelines for nutrition; they were replaced in August 1992 with the U.S. Department of Agriculture and U.S. Department of Health and Human Services' **Food Guide Pyramid: A Guide to Daily Food Choices.**

The revised Daily Food Guide reflects the knowledge accumulated in recent years about the need to cut down on fats and meats, and about the benefits of a diet high in vegetables, grains and fruits. Fortunately for all of us — and for our bones — a wide variety of delicious, healthy and readily-available food is high in calcium.

Below, you will find a summary of what nutrition experts consider

Food Guide Pyramid
A Guide to Daily Food Choices

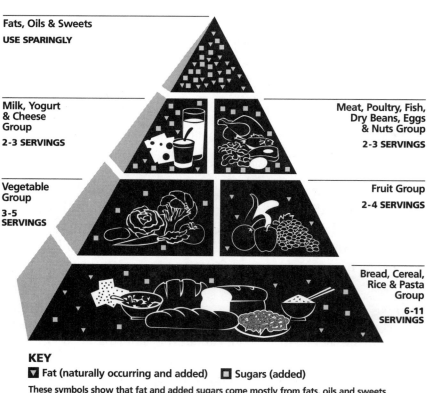

Fats, Oils & Sweets
USE SPARINGLY

Milk, Yogurt & Cheese Group
2-3 SERVINGS

Meat, Poultry, Fish, Dry Beans, Eggs & Nuts Group
2-3 SERVINGS

Vegetable Group
3-5 SERVINGS

Fruit Group
2-4 SERVINGS

Bread, Cereal, Rice & Pasta Group
6-11 SERVINGS

KEY
▼ Fat (naturally occurring and added)   ■ Sugars (added)

These symbols show that fat and added sugars come mostly from fats, oils and sweets, but can be part of or added to foods from the other food groups as well.
Source: U.S. Department of Agriculture/U.S. Department of Health and Human Services

a healthy diet. Remember that eating a variety of foods is important in a balanced diet, since each food is unique in its combination of nutrients. Suggestions for foods rich in calcium are listed in each of the food groups. Calcium content statistics are provided by the National Dairy Board and the National Dairy Council.

Food Choices for Healthy Eating

Bread, Cereal, Rice and Pasta Group

Recommended Daily: 6-11 Servings
Women and Older Adults: 6
Children, Teen Girls, Active Women, Most Men: 9
Teen Boys and Active Men: 11

Serving Size: 1 slice of bread, ½ cup cooked rice or pasta, ½ cup cooked cereal, 1 ounce ready-to-eat cereal

Calcium-Rich Choices: This food group offers little calcium, but is generally rich in iron, niacin and complex carbohydrates.

Vegetable Group

Recommended Daily: 3-5 Servings
Women and Older Adults: 3
Children, Teen Girls, Active Women, Most Men: 4
Teen Boys and Active Men: 5

Serving Size: ½ cup chopped raw or cooked vegetables, 1 cup leafy raw vegetables

Calcium-Rich Choices:

Food and Serving Size	Milligrams of Calcium
Broccoli, frozen, cooked, ½ cup	100
Turnip greens, fresh, cooked, ½ cup	99
Kale, frozen, cooked, ½ cup	90
Bok choy, fresh, cooked, ½ cup	79

Fruit Group

Recommended Daily: 2-4 Servings
Women and Older Adults: 2
Children, Teen Girls, Active Women, Most Men: 3
Teen Boys and Active Men: 4

Serving Size: 1 piece of fruit or a melon wedge, ¾ cup juice,
½ cup canned fruit, ¼ cup dried fruit

Calcium-Rich Choices: Fruits are not good sources of calcium, but
are rich in vitamins A and C.

Meat, Poultry, Fish, Dry Beans, Eggs and Nuts Group

Recommended Daily: 2-3 Servings
Women and Older Adults: 2, for a daily total of 5 ounces
Children, Teen Girls, Active Women, Most Men: 2, for a daily total
of 6 ounces
Teen Boys and Active Men: 3, for a daily total of 7 ounces

Serving Size: 2½ to 3 ounces cooked lean meat, poultry, fish; or
½ cup cooked beans, 1 egg or 2 tablespoons peanut butter all count
as 1 ounce of lean meat (about ⅓ of a serving)

Calcium-Rich Choices:

Food and Serving Size	Milligrams of Calcium
Sardines, with bones, 3 ounces	371
Salmon, with bones, 3 ounces	167
Tofu, 4 ounces	108
Shrimp, canned, 3 ounces	98
Beans, dried, cooked, 1 cup	90

Milk, Yogurt and Cheese Group

Recommended Daily: 2-3 Servings
Women and Older Adults: 2-3
Children, Teen Girls, Active Women, Most Men: 2-3
Teen Boys and Active Men: 2-3
(Note: Pregnant or lactating women and young adults to age 24
need 3 servings.)

Serving Size: 1 cup milk or yogurt, 1½ to 2 ounces cheese

Calcium-Rich Choices:

Food and Serving Size	Milligrams of Calcium
Vanilla milk shake, 11 ounces	457
Yogurt, plain, low fat, 1 cup	415
Ricotta cheese, part skim, ½ cup	337
Milk, skim, 1 cup	302
Milk, 1% low fat, 1 cup	300
Milk, 2% low fat, 1 cup	297
Milk, whole, 1 cup	291
Buttermilk, 1 cup	285
Milk, chocolate, 1 cup	280
Swiss cheese, 1 ounce	272
Monterey Jack cheese, 1 ounce	212
Mozzarella cheese, part skim, 1 ounce	207
Edam cheese, 1 ounce	207
Cheddar cheese, 1 ounce	204
Muenster cheese, 1 ounce	203
American cheese, pasteurized processed, 1 ounce	174
Blue cheese, 1 ounce	150
Ice milk, soft-serve, ½ cup	137
Pudding, chocolate, ½ cup	133
Sherbet, 2% fat, 1 cup	103
Ice cream, hard or soft, ½ cup	88

Combination Foods

The National Dairy Council offers the calcium content of some of your favorite multi-group foods:

Calcium-Rich Choices:

Food and Serving Size	Milligrams of Calcium
Cheese pizza, ⅛ of 15-inch pie	220
Macaroni and cheese, ½ cup	181
Spaghetti, meatballs and tomato sauce, 1 cup	124

To avoid excess fats and cholesterol, many dairy products come in fat-free and low-fat varieties. The National Dairy Council has these suggestions for adding more calcium to your diet:

- Prepare canned soups with milk instead of water.
- Add nonfat dry milk to soups, stews and casseroles.
- Add low-fat cheese to salads.

Lactose Intolerance

If you are one of those people who have difficulty digesting milk, it is most likely due to a lack of the intestinal enzyme *lactase*. This enzyme is necessary to break down *lactose*, or milk sugar. If someone who lacks this enzyme consumes products containing sufficient amounts of lactose, the result can be gastric disturbances like bloating, gas, cramps and diarrhea. However, there are still ways to consume dairy products and get your daily calcium.

Yogurt with bacteria cultures contains lactase, and can usually be eaten without discomfort, as can hard cheeses, in which the lactose has already been broken down by bacteria. Special dairy products, such as acidophilus milk, have been prepared with bacteria that contain lactase.

Your doctor may also recommend the use of over-the-counter enzyme products that break down lactose. These products usually come in liquid form, which can be added directly to milk, or in pill form to be taken before eating or drinking foods containing lactose.

Even if you can drink milk and eat any calcium-rich food you desire, certain other foods can rob you of your hard-earned calcium.

The Calcium Robbers

A certain amount of calcium is lost every day through the urine, feces and perspiration. This is commonly called *calcium excretion*. In addition, a number of foods and drinks can bind or react with calcium in a way that prevents the body from gaining the full benefit of a diligent daily intake. Some of these have been discussed in previous chapters, such as:

- *Fiber*, which hastens elimination and prevents adequate calcium absorption in the digestive tract. Fiber is usually a concern when ingested in excessive amounts or for persons who absorb calcium poorly in general.

- *Caffeine, salt, protein and carbonated beverages*, which can increase the excretion of calcium.

Other substances also interfere with the proper absorption of calcium. These foods contain phytates and oxalates, which combine with calcium and prevent its absorption through the digestive process. This lessens the amount of calcium that is *bioavailable*, meaning less calcium is in a form that your body can use. Experts recommend that you try to avoid having the following foods in the same meal as the foods you rely on for your calcium RDA:

- *Phytates:* Legumes, which are dried peas and beans.

- *Oxalates:* Endive, beets, parsley, spinach, amaranth greens, rhubarb, summer squash, peanuts, tea and cocoa.

As with fiber, foods containing phytates and oxalates need not be eliminated from the diet altogether — they pose a risk primarily to people who absorb calcium poorly, such as the elderly, or in people who fail to eat a well-balanced diet that contains a variety of foods.

Calcium Supplements

The best way to get your RDA of calcium is from your diet, because the foods you eat to reach your recommended calcium intake also provide other nutrients. A great number of people, however, do not get enough calcium from the foods they eat. Surveys and studies have shown that most of us are getting only about half of the calcium we need each day. In 1986, the U.S. Department of Agriculture conducted a survey that revealed the average woman gets just over 600 milligrams of calcium each day from her diet — far below the recommended minimum intake of 1,000 milligrams.

A number of options can help you get your much-needed daily

calcium. *Calcium supplements* are available as tablets, liquids or even antacids, and can be easily incorporated into your daily diet plan to ensure adequate calcium intake. When deciding which calcium supplement is right for you, there are several issues you must examine:

■ **Absorption:** In order for a calcium supplement to be most effective, it must be easily broken down and absorbed in the digestive tract. The National Osteoporosis Foundation recommends this easy test to check how readily a supplement will break down in the stomach:

Place the supplement in a glass of vinegar at room temperature. Let it sit for half an hour, stirring occasionally. If the tablet has broken down in the vinegar after 30 minutes, it should also do so in your stomach.

■ **Elemental calcium content:** In supplements, calcium is combined with a variety of other ingredients. The actual percentage of elemental calcium — the kind your body needs — is different in each type of supplement. As you will see in the chart that follows, the percentage of elemental calcium ranges from 40 percent to under 10 percent, depending on the type of supplement you choose.

■ **Side effects and drug interaction:** The most common negative side effects of calcium supplements are constipation, flatulence and irritation of the digestive tract. Some people may experience nausea. Calcium supplements interact with some prescription or over-the-counter drugs, so be sure to check with your pharmacist before you choose your supplements. Also, large amounts of calcium (in excess of 2,000 milligrams daily) may increase your risk for kidney stones if you have a personal or family history of that condition, and may actually increase bone loss.

Some forms of calcium — bone meal and dolomite — are not recommended by nutritionists. They may contain high levels of lead or other toxic metals. To be on the safe side, it is a good idea to discuss with your doctor the type and amount of calcium supplement that is appropriate for you.

How to Get the Most Out of Your Supplements

As discussed earlier, several types of food interfere with calcium absorption. In addition, supplements may also be more effective when taken at certain times of the day, and in certain dosages. Here are some important considerations when taking calcium supplements:

- **Do not take supplements along with high-fiber foods or laxatives,** which decrease calcium absorption.

- **Keep single doses to 500 to 600 milligrams or less.** Absorption increases when calcium is taken in smaller amounts more often.

- **Avoid taking calcium along with an iron supplement** because calcium interferes with the absorption of iron.

- **Some forms of calcium supplement should be taken with meals,** such as calcium carbonate and calcium phosphate, since they may be difficult to digest for people with low levels of stomach acid.

You need not plan your diet around calcium supplements, but keep these tips in mind to increase the effectiveness of your calcium intake. Be sure to drink plenty of liquids, and try to incorporate your supplement intake into your normal daily routine.

The chart on the next page describes several of the most common supplements available, and some of the characteristics of each.

CALCIUM SUPPLEMENT	% ELEMENTAL CALCIUM	COMMENTS	BRANDS/MILLIGRAMS CALCIUM PER TABLET
Calcium carbonate	40%	Best taken with meals. Not good for people with low stomach acid. Inexpensive. May cause gas, nausea or constipation.	Tums EX 300 mg Os-Cal 250 or 500 mg Caltrate 600 mg Chooz Gum 200 mg Alka-2 200 mg
Calcium lactate	13%	Contains lactose; not suitable for those who are lactose intolerant. More pills must be taken each day due to low calcium content.	Available in pill form of low dosage (under 100 mg)
Calcium gluconate	9%	Usually does not irritate stomach. More pills must be taken each day due to low calcium content.	Pill form, varying dosages
Calcium phosphate (diabasic)	30%	Taken with meals. Found in some calcium-fortified foods. Does not usually cause gas. Also provides phosphorus. Vitamin D added.	Di-Cal D capsules 117 mg Di-Cal D wafers 232 mg
Chelated calcium	Varies by brand	Manufacturers claim better absorption. Expensive. Solubility and percentage of elemental calcium vary by brand.	
Calcium citrate	21%	Good absorption. May be taken by those with low stomach acid. Expensive.	Citracal 200 mg

Calcium-Rich Recipes

For those who cannot get adequate calcium from dietary sources, supplements should strongly be considered. But if you think the only way to get dietary calcium is by drinking milk or eating yogurt or cottage cheese, you have a pleasant surprise coming!

Appetizers

Lite and Lean Nachos

A special preparation method results in nachos exceptionally low in fat but high in flavor.

6 6-inch corn tortillas
Vegetable oil spray
Salt
1 15-ounce can pinto beans, drained
3 ounces (¾ cup) shredded Cheddar cheese
2 small tomatoes, chopped
2 green onions, chopped
¼ cup plain yogurt

Cut each tortilla into 6 wedges, like a pie. Spread wedges in a single layer on cookie sheet. Spray with vegetable oil spray and sprinkle with salt. Bake at 375 degrees for about 5 minutes. Turn wedges over and sprinkle with salt. Bake for about 5 more minutes or until crispy. Mash pinto beans with a potato masher or fork, and heat thoroughly over medium heat, stirring occasionally. Spread tortilla chips on a heatproof platter; top with beans and cheese. Bake at 375 degrees for about 5 minutes, until cheese melts. Top with tomatoes, onions and yogurt.

Servings: 4
Calories per serving: 228
Calcium per serving: 282 mg

Seasoned Mozzarella Snacks

8 ounces part-skim mozzarella cheese
2 eggs
1 tablespoon nonfat milk
¾ cup dry bread crumbs
2 teaspoons Italian seasoning, crushed
2 teaspoons garlic powder
1½ tablespoons chopped parsley
¼ cup unsifted flour

Cut cheese into 24 1-inch-square cubes; set aside. In a pie pan beat eggs and milk. In another pie pan combine bread crumbs, Italian seasoning, garlic powder and chopped parsley. Place flour in a small bowl. Coat cheese cubes completely with flour, then egg mixture, and finally with bread crumbs. Repeat egg and bread crumb coatings. Place in a single layer on a plate, cover with foil, and refrigerate 2-3 hours or overnight. Preheat oven to 400 degrees. Place cheese cubes on a foil-lined baking sheet. Bake until crisp, 6-7 minutes. Let stand a few minutes before serving.

Servings: 12, 2 pieces each
Calories per serving: 82
Calcium per serving: 149 mg

Stuffed Bread Rolls

1 16-ounce loaf frozen bread dough
1 bunch Swiss chard
3 ounces (¾ cup) shredded Cheddar cheese
1 egg, beaten
2 tablespoons minced onion
1 tablespoon margarine
½ teaspoon garlic powder
2 tablespoons grated Parmesan cheese

Let bread dough thaw to room temperature according to package directions. Boil Swiss chard 15-20 minutes in covered pot with 1-2 inches water. Drain well and cool. Mix Swiss chard, Cheddar cheese, egg and onion. Cut dough in half. On lightly floured board, roll out dough into two 8-by-10-inch rectangles. Spread Swiss chard mixture over dough to within 1 inch of edges. Beginning with long side, roll up tightly. Lightly grease or spray bottom of a 9-by-13-inch pan. Place dough rolls in pan, seam down. Melt margarine and combine with garlic powder and Parmesan cheese; brush on top of rolls. Let rolls rise until tripled. Bake at 375 degrees for 25-30 minutes or until golden brown. Cut each roll into 12 slices.

Servings: 12, 2 slices each
Calories per serving: 154
Calcium per serving: 112 mg

Beverages

Tropical Teaser

1 cup pineapple juice
½ cup evaporated nonfat milk
⅓ cup instant nonfat dry milk
¼ teaspoon coconut extract or to taste
½ teaspoon rum extract or to taste
1 ripe medium banana, sliced
6 ice cubes

Pour pineapple juice and evaporated milk into blender, add dry milk and blend until smooth. Add extracts and sliced banana and blend again until smooth. Add ice cubes, one at a time, and blend on low speed after each one, until smooth. Blend on high until thick and frothy, about 30 seconds.

Servings: 3
Calories per serving: 129
Calcium per serving: 220 mg

Mocha Instant Breakfast

...with just enough caffeine to get you going in the morning!

¾ cup whole milk, very cold
¾ cup instant nonfat dry milk
½ teaspoon instant coffee
2 teaspoons cocoa
1 tablespoon sugar
pinch of salt
5 ice cubes

Blend liquid milk and dry milk in blender. Add coffee, cocoa, sugar and salt and blend until smooth. Add ice cubes, one at a time, and blend on low speed after each one, until smooth. Blend on high for 30 seconds, until thick and frothy.

Servings: 2
Calories per serving: 163
Calcium per serving: 391 mg

Berry Delight

Try making this refreshing drink with raspberries or strawberries, too.

1 cup plain yogurt
2 tablespoons boysenberry or strawberry jam or preserves
1 cup water
¾ cup frozen boysenberries, unsweetened

Blend ingredients in a blender until smooth, adding berries slowly.

Servings: 2, 1 cup each
Calories per serving: 151
Calcium per serving: 225 mg

Soups

Cream of Broccoli Soup

2 cups chicken broth
1 10-ounce package frozen chopped broccoli
4 tablespoons chopped parsley
1 medium onion, chopped
2 tablespoons lemon juice
2 cups evaporated nonfat milk
1 tablespoon cornstarch
Dash nutmeg
2 teaspoons garlic salt
$\frac{1}{4}$ teaspoon pepper
Parsley for garnish

Heat broth with broccoli, chopped parsley, onion and lemon juice to boiling. Cover and heat until broccoli is tender, according to package instructions. Remove vegetables from broth with a strainer and cool. Place vegetables in blender and add evaporated milk until blender is three-quarters full. Add cornstarch and blend until smooth. Slowly stir the vegetable-milk mixture, the rest of the evaporated milk, and the nutmeg, garlic salt and pepper into the broth. Heat over low flame until thickened, stirring constantly. Bring to a boil and boil lightly for 1 minute. Serve hot, garnished with parsley.

Servings: 5, 3/4 cup each
Calories per serving: 125
Calcium per serving: 355 mg

Hearty Bean Soup

Serve with a green salad and cornbread.

1 pound navy beans, washed and drained
3 quarts water
2 smoked ham hocks
1 10 $\frac{3}{4}$-ounce can beef broth
2 cloves garlic, minced

1 bay leaf
½ teaspoon salt
½ teaspoon pepper
2 cups mashed potatoes
3 medium onions, chopped
1½ cups diced celery, with leaves
¼ cup finely chopped parsley
2 cups diced carrot
2 tablespoons cider vinegar

Cover dry beans with water in soup pot, bring to a boil and boil 2 minutes. Remove from heat, cover and allow to stand for 1 hour. After 1 hour, add ham hocks, beef broth, garlic, bay leaf, salt and pepper to the beans. Simmer, covered, for 2 hours. Remove ham hocks; trim fat and bone from ham and cut ham into pieces; set aside. Add a little liquid from the soup to mashed potatoes to thin them until runny (this is done to prevent lumps). Stir potatoes, onions, celery, parsley, carrots and ham into the soup. Cover and simmer for another 1-1½ hours. Stir in cider vinegar. Let simmer a few minutes more.

Servings: 12 main-dish servings
Calories per serving: 200
Calcium per serving: 78 mg

Marvelous Meatless Chili

Great for leftovers, this low-calorie chili is one of our favorites.

1½ cups sliced carrot
1½ cups chopped onion
1½ cups chopped green pepper
1½ cups sliced celery
1 15-ounce can stewed tomatoes
1 15-ounce can tomato puree (or tomato sauce)
1 6-ounce can tomato paste
1 6-ounce can tomato juice
Juice of 1 lemon
2 15-ounce cans kidney beans, drained (reserve liquid)
1 15-ounce can chickpeas (garbanzo beans)

3 medium cloves garlic, minced
2-3 tablespoons chili powder
1 teaspoon sugar
1½ teaspoons dried basil
1 teaspoon salt
½ teaspoon pepper
½ teaspoon red pepper sauce

Heat cut-up vegetables in a large nonstick pot until just barely tender, stirring occasionally. Add rest of ingredients and mix well. If too thick, add reserved kidney bean juice. Cover and simmer for about 20 minutes. Do not overcook or vegetables will be mushy.

Servings: 16, ¾ cup each
Calories per serving: 122
Calcium per serving: 48 mg

Salads

Refreshing Fruit Salad

This unique fruit salad is sure to get rave reviews!

1 8-ounce package Neufchatel cheese, softened
1 cup cherry yogurt
1 tablespoon sugar
⅛ teaspoon vanilla
¼ teaspoon salt
1 16-ounce can pitted dark sweet cherries, drained
1 cup orange sections, cut in half
1 8-ounce can juice-packed crushed pineapple, drained
½ cup dried currants
Salad greens

Beat Neufchatel cheese in large mixing bowl until smooth. Beat in yogurt, sugar, vanilla and salt on low speed. Set aside 6-12 cherries for garnish. Stir remaining cherries, orange sections, pineapple and currants into cheese mixture. Pour into a 4½-cup mold or six individual molds. Freeze at least 8 hours. Remove mold(s) from freezer and let stand at room temperature until softened, about 45-60 minutes for large mold. Unmold on salad greens. Garnish with reserved cherries.

Servings: 6
Calories per serving: 265
Calcium per serving: 115 mg

Caesar Salad

Delightful with sourdough bread.

1 egg
3 tablespoons olive oil
¼ teaspoon garlic powder
1 cup cubed white bread, crust removed
1 medium clove garlic, crushed
¼ teaspoon dry mustard
½ teaspoon salt
¼ teaspoon ground pepper
2 tablespoons water
1½ teaspoons Worcestershire sauce
8 anchovy fillets, drained and chopped
1 large bunch romaine lettuce, torn
¼ cup grated Parmesan cheese
¼ cup crumbled blue cheese
2 tablespoons lemon juice

Warm cold egg by immersing in warm water. In a small saucepan, boil enough water to cover egg completely. Immerse egg in boiling water with spoon; remove from heat. Cover and let stand 30 seconds. Immediately cool egg in cold water to prevent further cooking. Heat 1 tablespoon of the olive oil and garlic powder in nonstick skillet. Add bread cubes and saute until browned, stirring often. Combine crushed garlic, mustard, salt, pepper, oil, water, Worcestershire sauce and anchovies in jar; cover and shake vigorously. Pour this dressing over lettuce in salad bowl, add cheeses and toss salad until it is well coated. Break egg into center of the salad. Pour lemon juice on top of egg and toss well. Add bread cubes, toss gently and serve immediately.

Servings: 6
Calories per serving: 136
Calcium per serving: 143 mg

Salmon Macaroni Salad

This salad is a complete meal and can be served as a main course or side dish.

1 12-ounce package salad macaroni (about 2¾ cups dry)
1 15-ounce can salmon
1½ cups cooked whole-kernel corn
1½ cups finely chopped bell pepper (red and/or green)
½ cup chopped onion
¾ cup chopped jicama
Salt and pepper to taste
⅔ cup diet mayonnaise
⅔ cup plain yogurt
Paprika

Cook macaroni according to package directions, omitting salt. Drain and cool. Drain salmon and break into chunks in large bowl. Add macaroni, corn, bell pepper, onion, jicama, salt and pepper, mixing well. Blend together mayonnaise and yogurt. Fold into salad ingredients. Place on salad plates lined with spinach leaves. Sprinkle with paprika.

Servings: 18, ¾ cup each
Calories per serving: 152
Calcium per serving: 74 mg

Entrees

Broccoli-stuffed Pasta

6 ounces (18-20) jumbo pasta shells
1 16-ounce bag frozen chopped broccoli, thawed
1 pound low-fat cottage cheese
8 ounces (2 cups) shredded part-skim mozzarella cheese
½ cup grated Parmesan cheese
1 tablespoon grated onion
½ teaspoon pepper
2 cloves crushed garlic or 1 teaspoon garlic powder
2 15½-ounce jars marinara sauce (or spaghetti sauce)

Cook pasta according to package directions. Drain. Combine broccoli, cottage cheese, 1½ cups mozzarella cheese, Parmesan cheese, onion, pepper and garlic. Fill shells with cheese-broccoli mixture. Spoon enough marinara sauce into bottom of 9-by-13-inch baking pan to cover bottom. Arrange shells in single layer; spoon remaining sauce over shells. Sprinkle rest of mozzarella cheese on top. Cover the pan with foil and bake at 375 degrees for 15 minutes. Remove the foil and bake for 15 more minutes, until heated thoroughly.

Servings: 6
Calories per serving: 437
Calcium per serving: 493 mg

Chicken Enchiladas

Even the strictest waist-watcher will enjoy this low-fat version of a favorite Mexican dish.

1½ chicken breasts, skinned
1¾ cups (14 fluid ounces) chicken broth, fat skimmed off
    (reserved from cooking chicken)
¼ cup cornstarch
1 28-ounce can enchilada sauce
1 teaspoon sugar

1 teaspoon chili powder
12 corn tortillas
2 cups plain yogurt
2 ounces ($\frac{1}{2}$ cup) shredded part-skim mozzarella cheese
2 ounces ($\frac{1}{2}$ cup) diced low-calorie processed Cheddar cheese
1 large onion, finely chopped
3 ounces ($\frac{3}{4}$ cup) shredded Cheddar cheese
3 ounces ($\frac{3}{4}$ cup) shredded Monterey Jack cheese
2 green onions, chopped

Cook chicken in water to cover until tender. Cool, then shred meat finely and discard bones. Reserve $1\frac{3}{4}$ cups broth. Dissolve cornstarch thoroughly in $\frac{1}{2}$ cup enchilada sauce. Pour remaining enchilada sauce into a saucepan; blend in cornstarch mixture, sugar and chili powder. Soften tortillas by wrapping them in stacks of six in moistened paper towels and then in foil. Seal foil tightly; heat in 250-degree oven for 15 minutes. Beat yogurt with a fork until smooth; add small amount of broth to it until runny. Add yogurt and remaining reserved broth to enchilada-sauce mixture. Heat and stir over low-medium flame, adding mozzarella and low-calorie Cheddar cheeses and heating until melted. Do not boil. To assemble enchiladas, unwrap warmed tortillas. Place on each some of the chicken, onion, Cheddar cheese and 1 tablespoon sauce. Roll and place seam side down in 9-by-13-inch baking pan. Top with sauce, using at least 2 cups. Sprinkle with Monterey Jack and remaining Cheddar. Bake at 350 degrees until cheese is melted and sauce is bubbly, about 25-30 minutes. Top with green onions.

Servings: 6
Calories per serving: 447
Calcium per serving: 617 mg

Oriental Omelet

9-10 ounces firm tofu, drained and finely cubed
3 eggs, lightly beaten
1 tablespoon soy sauce
$\frac{1}{4}$ teaspoon honey
1 tablespoon sesame oil

3 large fresh mushrooms, sliced
2 green onions, chopped

Combine first four ingredients in a large bowl and mix well. Heat oil in a large nonstick skillet. Add mushrooms and green onion, and saute 2-3 minutes, until slightly cooked. Add mushrooms and onions to tofu-egg mixture and stir. Pour mixture back into skillet and cook over low heat, lifting gently at sides to allow uncooked egg to flow underneath. When omelet is cooked, fold and serve.

Servings: 3
Calories per serving: 193
Calcium per serving: 149 mg

Pineapple Chicken

2 ounces sliced unsalted almonds
1 large onion, diced
2 12-ounce cans nonfat evaporated milk
1 4-ounce can sliced mushrooms
1 teaspoon salt
$\frac{1}{2}$ teaspoon pepper
$\frac{1}{8}$ teaspoon powdered ginger
1 16-ounce can unsweetened pineapple chunks, drained
2 teaspoons cornstarch
$2\frac{1}{3}$ cups cooked skinless chicken, cubed
4 cups cooked rice
Parsley

Brown almonds in nonstick skillet. Remove almonds and cook onion until tender. (Add a little water to pan, if needed.) To onion add all but $\frac{1}{2}$ cup of the milk, mushrooms, salt, pepper, ginger and pineapple. Stir over medium heat until hot. Add cornstarch to reserved milk and blend. Add chicken, almonds and cornstarch mixture to sauce and bring to a boil, stirring constantly. Boil 1 minute. Serve over rice. Garnish with parsley.

Servings: 6
Calories per serving: 457
Calcium per serving: 427 mg

Vegetables

Colorful Vegetable Bake

1 cup sliced carrots, fresh or frozen, thawed and drained
1½ cups sliced green beans, fresh or frozen, thawed and drained
1 14-ounce block firm tofu, drained
1 1-pound can whole tomatoes, drained
1 cup corn, fresh or frozen, thawed and drained
2 cloves garlic, minced
½ teaspoon salt
Dash of pepper
¼ cup slivered almonds

If fresh carrots and green beans are used, they will be crunchy unless partially precooked. Steam them for 5 minutes, if desired. Cut tofu into ½-inch cubes and quarter the canned tomatoes. Combine all ingredients except almonds in a large bowl and mix thoroughly. Transfer into greased 2-quart casserole. Top with almonds. Bake uncovered at 375 degrees until vegetables are cooked and tender, 30-40 minutes.

Servings: 12, ½ cup each
Calories per serving: 64
Calcium per serving: 69 mg

Spaghetti Squash Mozzarella

Spaghetti squash is a large oblong yellow summer squash that separates into spaghetti-like strands after it's cooked.

½ spaghetti squash, cut lengthwise
2 ounces (½ cup) shredded part-skim mozzarella cheese
1 tablespoon grated Parmesan cheese
3 tablespoons seasoned dry bread crumbs
1 teaspoon garlic powder
1 tablespoon chopped parsley

Clean out seeds from squash. Place squash, cut side down, in a pot with 2 inches water; cover and boil for 20 minutes. Completely scoop out strands of cooked squash into a bowl by running fork over inside. In another bowl combine remaining ingredients and mix well. Add this mixture to bowl with squash and blend. Place in casserole dish and bake uncovered at 350 degrees until slightly browned and cheese melts, about 20 minutes.

Servings: 8, ½ cup each
Calories per serving: 42
Calcium per serving: 82 mg

Broccoli Stir-fry

A classic Chinese dish.

1 pound broccoli
1 tablespoon vegetable oil
1 clove garlic, crushed
½ teaspoon salt
1 teaspoon rice wine or dry sherry
¼ teaspoon sugar
3 tablespoons chicken broth
¼ cup water

Rinse broccoli in cold water. Cut into 2-inch flowerets and slice stems ¼ inch thick. Heat oil in a nonstick skillet or wok over high heat for 30 seconds. Add broccoli stems and salt. Stir-fry for 30 seconds. Add broccoli flowerets. Stir-fry 1 minute. Add wine, sugar, broth and water. Reduce heat to medium-low and continue to stir-fry until water is almost gone. Serve hot.

Servings: 4, ½ cup each
Calories per serving: 53
Calcium per serving: 69 mg

Desserts

Almond Coffee Cake

1 cup sugar
⅓ cup margarine, softened
3 eggs
1½ teaspoons vanilla
1 12-ounce can almond filling
3 cups whole-wheat flour
2 teaspoons baking powder
½ cup nonfat dry milk
1½ teaspoons baking soda
½ teaspoon salt
1½ cups plain yogurt
7 tablespoons powdered sugar
2 teaspoons warm milk

Grease tube pan or Bundt cake pan. Beat sugar, margarine, eggs and vanilla in large mixing bowl on medium speed for about 2 minutes, scraping bowl occasionally. Blend in almond filling. Combine flour, baking powder, dry milk, baking soda and salt; blend into egg mixture alternately with yogurt. Pour batter into pan and bake in preheated oven at 350 degrees about 1 hour, until toothpick inserted near center comes out clean. Cool in pan about 15 minutes, then remove from pan. Mix powdered sugar and warm milk until smooth. Drizzle over cake.

Servings: 16
Calories per serving: 315
Calcium per serving: 141 mg

Cottage Cheesecake

Serve with fresh strawberries or other fruit topping.

Crust:
20 graham cracker squares
4 tablespoons margarine, softened
2 tablespoons sugar

Filling:
2 pounds low-fat cottage cheese, drained
¾ cup sugar
3 eggs, lightly beaten
1 teaspoon vanilla

Topping:
1 cup plain yogurt, drained of excess liquid. (If firm topping is
  desired, hang yogurt in triple-layered cheesecloth for
  1-2 hours to remove excess liquid.)
2½ tablespoons sugar
1½ teaspoons vanilla

To make pie crust, crush graham crackers with rolling pin, or in blender or food processor. Mix in margarine and sugar until fine crumbs are made. Press mixture into the bottom of a 9-inch spring-form pan. Bake at 350 degrees about 10 minutes.

To make the filling, blend cottage cheese, sugar, eggs and vanilla in blender or food processor until smooth. Pour into pie crust and bake at 350 degrees until firm, about 40 minutes.

To make the topping, blend yogurt, sugar and vanilla. Spread over baked cheesecake and let cool. Refrigerate before serving.

Servings: 12
Calories per serving: 245
Calcium per serving: 100 mg

Special Baked Apple

1 large apple
¼ teaspoon cinnamon
1 tablespoon packed brown sugar
1 cup plain yogurt

Core and slice apple; arrange in small casserole. Top with cinnamon and brown sugar. Bake uncovered at 375 degrees until tender, about 40 minutes. After 20 minutes, stir slices. Transfer slices to serving dishes and top each with ½ cup plain yogurt.

Servings: 2
Calories per serving: 164
Calcium per serving: 222 mg

CHAPTER 9

Great Beginnings: Raising Bone-Healthy Children

*A*ll parents want their children to grow up to be happy, healthy adults who live long and productive lives. The extent to which a parent can influence a child in this direction is limited, however. In the early years, before your children begin making many of their own choices about food and lifestyle, you can best help them establish their fundamental values concerning a healthy way of living.

Department of Health and Human Services studies have revealed a decline in the overall health of our children. In the past 30 years the percentage of obese children ages 6 to 11 has increased by more than 50 percent. Study after study shows that American children are less physically active than ever before, spending more time in passive activities. They are steadily increasing the hours they spend in front of the television set and decreasing the time engaged in creative play and exercise.

Up until the last decade or so, bone experts felt that peak bone mass was achieved between the ages of 25 and 35. The new school of thought is that trabecular bone, the more metabolically active form of bone that makes up much of the spine and the ends of long bones, actually reaches its peak mass much earlier — between the

195

ages of 15 and 20. Perhaps this fact, more than any other, empha-sizes the importance of a bone-friendly childhood. **The density of your child's bones at the time of peak bone mass is one of the two most important factors in determining whether your child will develop osteoporosis later in life.** The other factor is the rate at which bone is lost after peak bone mass is reached.

Two important aspects of raising physically healthy children are also crucial in maximizing their peak bone mass: diet and exercise. As parents, we know that we have precious few years in which we control these two elements of our children's good health. It all adds up to one inescapable conclusion: Our children will be more at risk for disease in their adult years if they lack proper diet and physical activity as youngsters. Whether your child becomes one of the osteo-porosis statistics later in life may well depend a great deal on what you teach your child today.

In this chapter you will learn how to help a healthy child achieve the greatest possible peak bone mass, how to get your child inter-ested in good nutrition and exercise, and how to deal with some of the pitfalls of raising a bone-healthy child in this age of fast food and television.

B. Lawrence Riggs, M.D., professor of Medical Research, Mayo Medical School, served as Board President of the National Osteoporosis Foundation from 1990 through 1992. When asked what parents can do to help their children prevent osteoporosis, Dr. Riggs responded: "The three areas that should receive the most attention are nutrition, physical activity and, in young women, menstrual irregularity. Nutrition is an area in which we could see major improvements." With that in mind, let's take a look at the role that childhood nutrition plays in the prevention of adult diseases, particularly osteoporosis.

Nutrition and Your Child

A child does not have to be overweight to have a dietary problem. Your child may be of average weight, but have a diet that contains too few vital nutrients and too many unnecessary or even harmful ingredients. For example, you may be surprised to learn that children and teenagers can have dangerously high cholesterol levels — and if that child's family is predisposed to cardiovascular disease, the chances of the child developing a serious health problem early in his or her adult life are greatly increased.

Sound nutrition is of particular importance in the prevention of osteoporosis. A significant percentage of bone is made up of calcium, and calcium must come from the foods we eat. In the teenage years, when the body is building the most bone it will ever have, the diet is probably as nutritionally poor as at any time during life. "Nutritional factors such as high protein and high meat intake, as well as excessive consumption of diet sodas, are perhaps detrimental to bone," says Dr. Riggs. Yet hamburgers, french fries and soft drinks are the staples of the young American diet. Unfortunately, these are not foods that contribute significantly to growing and maintaining healthy bones.

So what is good for young bodies in their peak bone formation years? "You just can't make bone without adequate calcium," says Dr. Riggs. "If you don't have enough calcium, you are not going to have a skeleton of maximal size." Surveys show that children are not getting the calcium they need to build bones — recent studies indicate that about one-third of children under the age of five are getting only about 75 percent of their recommended daily calcium intake. Remember — the lower the calcium intake, the lower the peak bone mass; the lower the peak bone mass, the greater the risk of osteoporosis later in life.

C. Conrad Johnston, Jr., M.D., professor of Medicine and Director of the Division of Endocrinology and Metabolism at Indiana University School of Medicine, conducted studies on young identical twins to determine the effect of calcium intake on bone density. Dr. Johnston and his associates found that those children who significantly increased their daily calcium above the RDA for their age showed an increase in bone mass when compared with their twins, who did not take additional calcium. Based on data from studies such as Dr. Johnston's, some osteoporosis experts feel that the RDA for calcium may be too low, especially for children.

Designing a Bone-Healthy Diet for Kids

How can you make sure your child gets enough calcium? Here are some guidelines you may find helpful:

1. Provide a well-rounded diet that does not entirely exclude your child's favorite foods. The quickest way to encourage a nutrition rebellion is to make your child feel deprived. Healthy eating should not be presented as punishment or personal sacrifice, but rather as something good we do for ourselves.

Get your children involved in choosing healthy foods. Take them to the grocery store with you, or perhaps prepare a list of "yes" foods from which they can choose healthy foods for themselves.

The U.S. Department of Agriculture's "Guide to Daily Food Choices" provides a guideline for your child's nutritional needs.

	Children	Teen Girls	Teen Boys
Calories per day	2,200	2,200	2,800
Servings of:			
Bread group	9	9	11
Vegetables	4	4	5
Fruits	3	3	4
Milk group	2-3	3	3
Meat group	2	2	3

For a full description of the food groups and serving sizes, see Chapter Eight.

2. Limit your child's intake of saturated fats, salt, meat, sugary snacks and carbonated soft drinks. Many low-fat and low-salt processed foods are popping up on the supermarket shelves — you just have to look for them and be a label-reader. Some varieties of cookies and other snack foods are targeting the more health-conscious consumer, so be on the lookout for ways to lower your children's intake of fats, sugars, salt and carbonated drinks, as well as limiting meat consumption to the recommended number of servings per day.

3. Encourage your child to eat and drink calcium-rich foods. The recommended dietary allowance for children ages 1 through 10 is 800 milligrams per day; for adolescents and young adults ages 11 through 24, the RDA is 1,200 milligrams per day. As mentioned earlier, however, a great number of children are not getting their RDA of calcium, and even fewer adolescents get the calcium they need each day. Some experts feel that the RDAs are too low, and research data indicates that bone density can be significantly increased by adding calcium to the diet.

A wide variety of foods and drinks that are high in calcium appeal to most kids. Milkshakes, frozen yogurt, cheese and chocolate milk are all great sources of calcium. Take a look at the list below — aren't these some of your children's favorite foods?

	Serving Size	Milligrams of Calcium
Vanilla milkshake	11 ounces	457
Frozen yogurt, fruit-flavored	8 ounces	240
Skim milk	8 ounces	302
Whole milk	8 ounces	291
Vanilla ice milk, soft-serve	8 ounces	274
Vanilla ice milk, hard	8 ounces	176
Cheddar cheese	1 ounce	204
Cheese pizza	⅛ of a 15-inch pie	220
Macaroni and cheese	4 ounces	181

4. Don't bring the "bad stuff" into the house. It's considerably easier to say "no" if the high-fat, high-salt junk food isn't sitting right there in the pantry. Children who constantly see these types of food at home may get the message that they are dietary staples rather than occasional treats.

5. Promote a healthy self-image in your child. This can be a challenge, especially with teenagers. Accent their positive traits, acknowledge their efforts and express your appreciation often. Ask for your child's opinion and suggestions on how the family can lead a more healthful lifestyle. Everyone, including children, needs to have some sense of control. Avoid negative comments that can damage your child's sense of self-worth and self-esteem. Try not to associate being a "good" kid with eating habits such as cleaning the plate. Self-image problems can lead to eating disorders and radical diets, and cause serious damage to growing bodies and minds.

6. Set a good example. It is pretty hard to convince your child to eat a well-balanced meal when your dinner consists of a candy bar and a soft drink. Children like explanations, and "because I said so" will work for only so long when it comes to good nutritional habits. Your kids may rebel against what you want them to do, but if you set a good example, they will see that you really believe in what you're asking them to do.

To give you a start on including tasty but calcium-rich foods in your child's diet, recipes with kid-appeal are provided at the end of this chapter.

Building Strong Bones with Exercise

Exercise is an essential partner to good nutrition for a healthy childhood. Physical activity is so natural to most children that a little encouragement and participation on your part will go a long way.

The right amount of physical activity is very important if your child is to attain the greatest possible peak bone mass. Too little exercise means that bone mass will never reach its full potential; too much exercise can lead to conditions that harm bone, such as menstrual dysfunction, as well as to deficiencies in the nutrients that build a strong skeleton.

To help young bodies achieve maximum peak bone mass, most experts recommend that parents encourage normal physical play that includes a variety of activities. Sheri Butler, M.A., exercise physiologist and Fitness Manager of the Peggy and Philip B. Crosby Wellness Center in Winter Park, Florida, stresses the importance of parental interaction. "Parents need to be involved in their children's physical fitness. Beginning with infants, we recommend that mothers and fathers engage in such activities as massaging the child's limbs. As children get older, parents can participate in the active play of toddlers and young children. Tune in to their cues. The children will usually let you know what type of physical play they are interested in — games of 'tag' and just running and jumping are great physical activities for children this age."

For these younger children, try games of "follow the leader" — taking turns being the leader, so that everyone gets a chance to exercise those leadership abilities. Vary the movements during your turn to provide different exercises. Swing your arms, stretch and bend your body and your imagination. How about creating an obstacle course — think safety first — that includes crawling, climbing, running and jumping actions? Activities like these can entertain children up to eight or nine years old, and you are interacting with your child on an important level.

Older children are usually ready to get into more rough-and-tumble play. At this age they often become more interested in sports. High-impact activities are fine for this age group: running, gymnastics, basketball, soccer — all are great exercises that help build bone mass. Butler has a word of caution for parents regarding their children and sports, however: "Parents should be certain that they do not push a child into a sport for which the child is not physically suited."

Butler also indicates that it is important not to overstress young bones. "Young people under the age of 18 have strong muscles, but the long bones such as the femur in the thigh have sensitive growth plates at each end. Weight-training and resistance exercises are fine, but rather than pile on excessive weight, they should use more repetitions and correct form for a healthier workout."

Set a good example: Turn off the television set and just get active with your child. Make physical activity a way of life for your whole family. Walk, ride bicycles, throw a ball around or whatever you all can safely do together. You do not have to be a world-class athlete to give your child three most precious gifts: a love for exercise, healthy bones and your undivided attention.

Menstrual Irregularities

As important as getting enough exercise, perhaps even more so, is avoiding excessive exercise in children. A young person who exercises heavily but does not provide his or her body with the needed nutrients can quickly develop health problems, including loss of bone mass. In young female athletes, a disturbance of the menstrual cycle called *amenorrhea* — a cessation of menstruation — can cause a significant decrease in bone mass.

Researchers are finding that bone loss in premenopausal women may be more common than has been assumed in the past. While considerable research has shown that young women with amenorrhea suffer premenopausal bone loss, some experts are currently studying the negative effects that other menstrual disturbances have on bone mass.

Drastic menstrual dysfunction in young women is most often the result of excessive physical exercise, such as marathon training, and eating disorders such as anorexia nervosa. The belief is that bone loss occurs as a result of the decrease in estrogen attributable to abnormally low levels of body fat.

Other menstrual disturbances currently under study may simply be manifested by irregular periods, and can be caused by problems within the various organs, glands and hormones that affect the menstrual cycle. Decreased production of various hormones — estrogen, progesterone or even androgens — can all affect the menstrual cycle and result in bone loss.

"Young women with menstrual irregularities have lower bone mass than girls with regular periods," says Dr. Riggs. "While we are not quite to the point of recommending hormone intervention for these young women, more data on this issue may indicate that hormone therapy could be used to treat these irregularities and slow the resulting bone loss. The therapy would be used on an interim basis until the menstrual cycle continues to be regular."

So here we have one more way to protect your children's healthy bones: Be alert to irregularities in your daughter's menstrual cycle, and encourage her to report any disturbances in the normal cycle to you or to her physician. Many teenagers feel that their mothers are prying into personal matters when they ask questions about their daughters' menstrual cycle. Make your reasons for asking clear to your daughter, and encourage her to talk to her doctor if she feels uncomfortable mentioning such problems to you.

Finally, consider passing this book along to older teenage children — especially girls — who need to learn early in life how to prevent osteoporosis. Young adults often feel impervious to injury, sickness and physical disability, but a little basic training may do more long-term good than you think.

As has been mentioned throughout this book, prevention is the most effective way to manage osteoporosis. Compared to many other aspects of parenting, helping your children build and maintain strong bones is a breeze — and it's an effort that will pay benefits to your children throughout their lifetime.

Calcium-Rich Recipes for Kids

Old-Fashioned Hot Cocoa

5 tablespoons sugar
⅓ cup cocoa
¼ teaspoon salt
1½ cups water
4½ cups whole milk
1 cup instant nonfat dry milk
½ teaspoon mint extract (optional)

Mix sugar, cocoa and salt in a 2-quart saucepan. Add water. Heat to boiling, stirring constantly. Boil and stir for 2 minutes. Stir in liquid milk and then slowly add dry milk, stirring continuously. Heat thoroughly but do not boil. Stir in extract, if desired. Just before serving, beat with a hand beater until foamy.

Servings: 6, 1 cup each
Calories per serving: 202
Calcium per serving: 365 mg

Garden Burrito

1 8-inch flour tortilla
½ cup canned, drained pinto beans
1 cup shredded lettuce
1 tomato, chopped
1 tablespoon chopped onion
2 ounces (½ cup) shredded Cheddar or Monterey Jack cheese
Salsa to taste

Warm flour tortilla in oven or microwave. Mash beans with potato masher or fork and cook over medium heat, stirring occasionally. Spread beans on tortilla. Top with lettuce, tomato, onion, cheese and salsa.

Servings: 1
Calories per serving: 527
Calcium per serving: 551 mg

Michigan Meatloaf

2 pounds ground round beef
2 eggs
1 cup nonfat dry milk
1 medium onion, diced
½ cup Italian-style bread crumbs
2 teaspoons salt
½ teaspoon garlic powder

Blend all ingredients well; form into a loaf. Bake in loaf pan or roasting pan, covered, at 350 degrees for about 1 ½ hours.

Servings: 1
Calories per serving: 212
Calcium per serving: 106 mg

Turkey Taco Casserole

8 6-inch corn tortillas
1¾ pounds ground turkey
1 onion, chopped
2 cloves garlic, pressed
1½ teaspoons chili powder
¼ teaspoon ground cumin
¼ teaspoon thyme
¼ teaspoon salt
½ teaspoon oregano

1 pound Monterey Jack
　cheese, shredded
6 eggs
2 cups nonfat milk
1 cup plain yogurt
3 tomatoes, chopped
3 cups shredded lettuce
Olives (optional)
Salsa (optional)

Line greased 9-by-13-inch baking dish with tortillas, tearing to fit and putting in two layers. In large skillet, brown turkey and onion, draining off fat. Add garlic, chili powder, cumin, thyme, salt and oregano. Pour into baking dish. Top with cheese. In bowl, beat eggs with milk and pour over ingredients in baking dish. Bake at 350 degrees for 1 hour, until custard sets. While still warm, spread with yogurt, then tomatoes, lettuce and olives, if desired. Pass salsa at table, if desired.

Servings: 12
Calories per serving: 378
Calcium per serving: 437 mg

Frozen Orange Yogurt

This is as good as the soft-serve kind, and easy to make at home.

1 3-ounce package orange-flavored gelatin
¾ cup sugar
1 cup water
1 cup orange juice
2 cups plain yogurt
1 cup evaporated whole milk, chilled

Also needed:
2 chilled metal bowls (2 sizes)
Chilled beaters

Combine gelatin, sugar and water in saucepan. Boil, stirring constantly, until sugar and gelatin are dissolved. Remove from heat and cool to room temperature (about 30 minutes). Stir in orange juice and yogurt. Pour into 9-by-13-inch pan. Freeze, stirring occasionally, until partially frozen, 2-3 hours. Spoon into chilled large bowl. Beat with chilled beaters until very smooth. In a smaller chilled bowl, whip milk until stiff. Fold whipped milk into yogurt mixture. Spoon into bowl or freezer container; cover and freeze until firm, 3-4 hours.

Servings: 9, 1 cup each
Calories per serving: 181
Calcium per serving: 168 mg

Frozen Peach Pops

A light, summery treat ... good any time of the year!

20 ounces frozen sweetened peaches
Reserved peach juice from frozen peaches
    (if unsweetened peaches are used,
    add 4 tablespoons sugar to juice)
1 envelope unflavored gelatin
2 cups plain yogurt

Also needed:
12 3-ounce paper cups
12 wooden ice cream sticks

Thaw peaches completely. Press thoroughly to remove all juice. Place drained juice (and sugar, if used) in a saucepan and sprinkle with gelatin. Cook over low heat, stirring until gelatin dissolves. Blend peaches, yogurt and juice with gelatin in a blender until smooth. Place cups in a baking pan and fill each with fruit mixture. Cover each cup with waxed paper; make a slit in the paper over the center of each cup and insert a stick for each pop. Freeze until firm. Run warm water on outside of cup to loosen it from pop before serving.

Servings: 12 pops
Calories per serving: 73
Calcium per serving: 70 mg

CHAPTER 10

Injury Prevention: Avoiding Falls and Fractures

A substantial number of injuries experienced by older adults are the result of taking a fall. In a typical year, about one-third of people over the age of 75 will experience a fall, with about one in every three of those accidents causing at least temporary disability. For someone whose bones are weakened by osteoporosis, the injury from a fall can be devastating. But many falls can be prevented with simple and inexpensive precautions.

Where and when do you suppose that elderly people fall most often? In a strange environment? No; research published by the National Institute on Aging indicates that the majority of falls — over 50 percent — occur in or around the home, and 75 percent of these happen in the bedroom or bathroom. While stumbling around in the dark, you say? Wrong again; most falls occur during the daytime.

Certain aspects of life — some avoidable, some unavoidable — are known to increase the risk of falling. Many of these factors more commonly affect older people. They include:

■ Medications, like sedatives and sleeping pills

■ Arthritis in the legs or hips

■ Impaired vision, particularly depth perception

- Weakened muscles and poor balance
- Parkinson's disease
- Decreased coordination and slowed reflexes
- Hazards in the home environment

This chapter examines these hazards in detail, in order to help you make two important aspects of your life more resistant to accidents and falls: your physical self and your home environment.

Taking Care of Yourself — Step One in Preventing Accidents

We all want to live as long as possible, but longevity has its trade-offs. Physical and mental changes that occur over time can make it harder to keep ourselves healthy and safe. As we age, we may occasionally need help getting to sleep, or develop conditions that make walking difficult, such as painful arthritis. Older adults often do not get the physical activity and proper nutrition they need to be strong and flexible. All of these conditions can lead to injury from falls.

Though many changes in ourselves are related to aging, not all problems can be blamed on "just getting old." A symptom such as loss of balance, poor eyesight or lack of coordination may actually be an indication of a treatable condition. For example, something as simple and easily treated as an ear infection or wax buildup may cause loss of balance. Don't ignore a change in the way you feel or in the functioning of your body because you think it is merely a result of your age — tell your doctor when physical changes occur.

Most older adults and those concerned with their care can do a great deal to help reduce their odds of taking a fall. The suggestions most often made by experts are:

1. **Review your medications**. Many prescription and over-the-counter medications can produce dizziness, light-headedness and drowsiness. Cold and allergy medications, pain relievers, muscle relaxants — all may include ingredients that make us feel unsteady on our feet. If you aren't sure of the side effects of any drug you're taking,

ask your doctor and/or pharmacist. Check to see whether another medication — or a smaller dosage of the same drug — will treat the symptoms without causing side effects that contribute to your risk of falling. Your medications' effects can continue for a number of hours after you take them. Drugs that remain in the body a short period of time may be preferable to those that remain in the system longer.

If you are taking sedatives, tranquilizers or sleeping pills, be especially alert to the fact that these types of drugs increase your risk of falling.

2. Have your eyes and ears checked regularly. Impaired vision, especially depth perception, is a common complaint as we get older. Small problems with your eyesight can cause you to miss subtle visual clues that could help prevent stumbling. Even if you already wear contact lenses or eyeglasses, your vision should be checked regularly.

The inner ear is the site of the *semicircular canals*, which control the sense of balance. These canals are filled with fluid. As your head moves, the fluid moves also, pressing against delicate nerve endings that let your body know in which direction the head is turning. This, in turn, helps maintain equilibrium. A number of factors can upset this delicate system; some are as simple as a wax buildup in the ear. Having your ears checked regularly is a good way to help preserve your sense of balance.

3. Maintain an appropriate level of physical activity. Staying physically active helps improve balance, coordination, flexibility and muscle strength — real assets in fall prevention. Check with your doctor about which forms of exercise are safe and beneficial for you. These may include swimming, walking or riding a stationary cycle. Do not start a new exercise program without an okay from your doctor; depending on your physical condition, it may be that you should exercise only under the supervision of a physical therapist or other exercise professional.

4. Avoid alcohol. Alcohol affects equilibrium and coordination and has an intensifying effect on some medications, such as sedatives and sleeping pills. If you drink alcohol, ask your doctor about its effect on any drugs you are taking.

5. Eat regularly and maintain a healthy diet. Most of us get quite woozy if we don't eat when and what we should. Changes in the glucose (blood sugar) level can result in faintness or an overall weak feeling. See Chapter Eight for more details on a healthy diet.

6. Don't get up too fast after eating or resting. Your blood pressure falls during these times, and if you rise too quickly you may feel lightheaded or wobbly.

7. Don't be afraid to ask for help if you need it. If you feel dizzy, faint or weak, sit down. Ask for a responsible person's assistance if you need to call a friend or caregiver to help you get home.

8. Don't rule out the use of walking support. Walkers and canes can add stability on the days when you are feeling unsteady, or when surfaces are icy or wet. A slight loss of mobility is far preferable to taking a fall that may land you in the hospital or in bed for weeks.

9. Take note of your footwear. Wear low-heeled, rubber-soled shoes that provide solid support for the foot and ankle. Avoid walking around in socks or hose, which can slip on smooth floors, or in shoes or slippers with smooth soles, or in sandals or scuffs that do not fit securely on the foot. If you have foot problems, see your orthopedic doctor or podiatrist. Have a professional treat bunions and corns that keep you from wearing supportive shoes that fit properly.

10. Teach yourself the safe way of performing everyday tasks. Older muscles and bones are less forgiving. We can no longer get away with performing routine movements in a haphazard manner. To avoid injury, it may be wiser in the long run to hire someone to do the more strenuous chores around the house, particularly things that require a ladder.

In the examples pictured on page 212, you will see the safe — and unsafe — way to perform a number of activities. Take note of the positioning of the body in the "Do" illustrations. Practice these movements, and refer back to the illustrations as often as necessary. Make yourself familiar and comfortable with the forms of movement that reduce strain and decrease the risk of injury.

Also talk to your doctor about the movements and activities that are most likely to cause spontaneous fractures of the spine and other osteoporotic fracture sites.

Taking Care of Your Environment — Step Two in Preventing Accidents

As many as half of all falls are due to hazards in the environment, especially in one's own home. While you may not be able to stumble-proof the world, you can certainly do a great deal to decrease the risk of accidents in your own home. Here are some of the most commonly recommended ways of making your environment more fall-resistant:

1. Provide Adequate Lighting Throughout Your Home. Hallways, porches, basements and stairways are some of the most poorly lit areas of the home. If you have difficulty focusing in dim lighting, use higher wattage light bulbs. Make sure light switches are easily accessible, and consider replacing overhead pull-cord switches with wall-mounted switches that can be used without risking your balance.

Keep night lights in your bedroom, bathroom and hallway — and use them every night. Even younger people are unsteady when they get up in the middle of the night, so don't take a chance on stumbling in the dark when a fixture that costs a few dollars can light the way for you.

2. Remove Hazards From Your Floors. Avoid using throw rugs, since they may bunch up easily and often curl on the ends. Use non-skid rug backing to anchor all of your rugs firmly to the floor, especially at the edges. Consider using non-skid strips instead of rugs

Performing Everyday Tasks the Safe Way

DO	DON'T	DO	DON'T

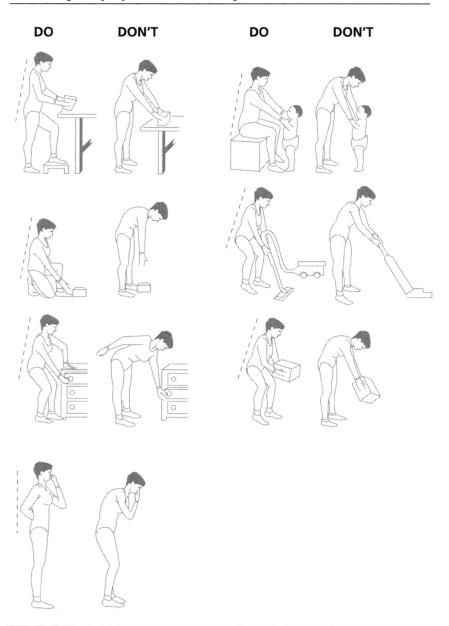

Simple daily activities can be done in ways that help prevent fractures. Take special note of the body positions in the DO illustrations above, and avoid those actions in the DON'T illustrations.

on stairs. If your stairs are carpeted, keep both the stairs and the carpeting in good repair, and have worn or frayed areas repaired immediately. Make sure handrails on stairs and porches are sturdy and well secured. Use non-skid mats or carpeting rather than rugs in bathrooms and kitchens, where floors are apt to get wet.

Clear your traffic areas of clutter, with electrical cords and telephone wires tucked away out of your path. Keep safety in mind when arranging furniture — position as many pieces as possible along the walls; furniture in the center of a room presents an obstacle course to foot traffic. Try to resist the urge to rearrange your furniture — it takes everyone a while to become familiar with a new layout, and increases the risk of a collision.

Avoid slippery surfaces. Wipe up spills as soon as they happen, and don't walk on wet floors — there are few things that can't wait until the floor is dry. Avoid the use of glossy waxes and polished types of ceramic tile and marble.

3. Prevent accidents in the bedroom and bathroom. Place your telephone, eyeglasses and a light switch within easy reach of the bed. Make sure to keep a night light on every night. Since many older adults have trouble adjusting from bright light to dim, provide adequate lighting in all rooms during the day.

Bathrooms must have adequate daytime light and a night light as well. Have grab bars installed in the shower and appropriately located near the toilet. Use non-skid mats rather than area rugs, and apply non-skid adhesive strips to the floor of the tub and shower. If you have trouble getting out of the tub, investigate specially-made seats that are placed in the bathtub to make getting in and out less awkward.

Be careful when using bath oils or bubble bath that may make the tub even more slippery. When you can comfortably do so, pick up small pieces of bar soap that drop off while bathing.

Use caution when cleaning tubs and toilets — determine the safest and most comfortable position in which you can accomplish these tasks.

A number of companies market products specifically designed to make life simpler and safer for older adults or persons with restrictive conditions like osteoporosis and arthritis. Check the appendix for a list of companies offering catalogs.

In the area of home safety, it often seems that the little things get in the way most often. The simple, inexpensive steps above can protect you and your family from injury. Take time to examine your home and yard for hazards that may have gone undetected. Take extra care protecting the most valuable thing in your home — you.

Getting Help:
Resources for Assistance
and Information

*R*ecent attention to the health issues of women and the elderly has many benefits. One of these is the increasing number of government and private programs dedicated to osteoporosis support and education. Special committees within the House of Representatives and the Senate have been formed to study the needs of the aging population. In the private sector, more and more hospitals and other organizations are establishing support groups and information sources for women and the elderly.

This appendix provides you with a list of valuable resources for what should be your continuing quest for information on osteoporosis. You are encouraged to spread your new-found knowledge. The next time you are at a family gathering or among friends, look around. The lives of as many as half of your female loved ones — your mother, sisters, cousins, daughters and granddaughters — will eventually be touched by osteoporosis. You can be a catalyst for change, however. You can help others become educated in ways of preventing osteoporosis, and help them recognize aspects of their own lives that increase the risk of osteoporosis.

The vast majority of the agencies, organizations and programs listed on the following pages offer their information and services free of charge. It costs you little or nothing to receive the knowledge and support that these resources offer, but the benefits may truly change your life and the lives of those you love.

This is by no means a complete list of the many resources available throughout the country. You will often find that one contact leads to another, and that a number of government and public organizations work in conjunction with other groups. Pick and choose those that best fit your needs, and you will soon compile an entire network of support and information sources.

National Osteoporosis Foundation
1150 17th Street, NW
Washington, DC 20036-4603

Founded in 1986, the National Osteoporosis Foundation is the country's leader in information on osteoporosis. Not only is it an excellent resource for individuals, it also helps physicians, hospitals and other health care professionals keep in touch with the latest data on osteoporosis prevention, treatment and research. Individual memberships are available, and include a subscription to their excellent newsletter (published quarterly) and updates on pertinent legislation and medical news.

Government and Public Organizations and Programs

National Institutes of Health
Public Information Office
9000 Rockville Pike
Bethesda, MD 20892

The NIH Public Information Office will answer questions about NIH projects, including the Women's Health Initiative, and has a number of informative publications available to the public.

National Institute on Aging
9000 Rockville Pike
Bethesda, MD 20892

Part of the National Institutes of Health, this organization can provide information on health issues that affect aging Americans. Write for information.

National Institute of Arthritis and Musculoskeletal and Skin Diseases
9000 Rockville Pike
Bethesda, MD 20892

This organization maintains a list of helpful documents available through a number of sources. Write for information.

U.S. Consumer Product Safety Commission
Washington, DC 20207

This agency can provide information on making your home and environment safer. One booklet that may be especially helpful is "Safety for Older Consumers: Home Safety Checklist," available at no charge. Send a postcard to the address above.

U.S. House Select Committee on Aging
300 New Jersey Avenue, SE
Room 712, Annex 1
Washington, DC 20515

U.S. Senate Special Committee on Aging
Dirksen Office Building
Washington, DC 20510

The House of Representatives and the Senate have members serving on special committees that focus on the needs of the aging population. Write for information on legislation affecting the elderly.

Local Offices

Social Security Administration
State, County or City Area
  Agencies
State Colleges and Universities
Public Libraries

Check the government pages of your phone book for departments and agencies that provide information and services for the elderly. Many offer special programs for the aging, such as transportation assistance, group activities and counseling on such issues as nutrition and health care. Many of these programs are free — available for the asking.

Some of the larger state universities have departments devoted to the study of aging (gerontology), and can be a valuable source of information.

The public library and its reference librarian may be one of America's best — and most underutilized — assets. These institutions have the world at their fingertips, and can provide you with mountains of information on virtually any topic at ABSOLUTELY NO CHARGE. Get to know your library.

Private Organizations

American Association of Retired Persons (AARP)
1909 K Street, NW
Washington, DC 20049

This huge organization has a strong voice in legislation affecting the older American, including health issues. With more than 30 million members and growing, it is a force to be reckoned with. Write or call to inquire about membership and/or some of the publications available on a wide spectrum of health issues.

Personal and Home Products

These companies offer catalogs of products that can help you prevent falls and other injuries. These references are provided for information only, and should not be considered an endorsement of any products offered for sale by these companies.

AfterTherapy Catalog
1-800-634-4351
Easy Living
1-800-645-5272
Enrichments for Better Living
1-800-323-5547
Independent Living Aids Catalog
1-800-537-2118
J.C. Penney Easy Dressing
  Fashions
1-800-222-6161

Hospitals and Support Groups

A great many hospitals have women's health centers and a variety of support groups, including those for osteoporosis patients. Most support groups are self-help organizations, often led by a hospital staff member or affiliated physicians. They are committed to education, emotional support and the sharing of ideas and resources. According to a survey conducted by the National Osteoporosis Foundation, most participants in osteoporosis groups are women who have osteoporosis, but over half the support groups responding to the survey also included members who were family, friends or caregivers of people with the disease.

Support groups are sometimes formed by private individuals, without affiliation with a hospital or other organized institution.

Most support groups, regardless of affiliation, offer networking opportunities for members to meet other people with osteoporosis, to discuss special challenges facing osteoporotic individuals, and to gain knowledge from speakers — often medical specialists, nutritionists and exercise professionals.

To find an osteoporosis support group near you, contact the large hospitals in your area, check your phone book under "Associations" or similar headings, or ask your doctor or community senior center if they know of any such groups in the area. If you are unable to locate a support group and would like information on starting one, contact the National Osteoporosis Foundation.

Glossary

Amenorrhea: The abnormal cessation of menstruation.

Anabolic steroids: The family of drugs derived from the male hormone testosterone. They stimulate the body's metabolic process of muscle and bone growth in males, and are responsible for the greater body size and strength of men as compared to women.

Androgens: The male sex hormones, the primary of which is testosterone.

Anti-resorptive agent: Osteoporosis intervention that works by repressing the osteoclasts, therefore reducing the amount of bone broken down.

Appendicular skeleton: The bones of the limbs.

Biochemical marker: A chemical found in the blood or urine that is indicative of certain biological processes, such as bone remodeling.

Bisphosphonates: Also called **diphosphonates**, an osteoporosis intervention that belongs to a class of compounds that are adsorbed (attracted and retained) to the calcium phosphate crystalline structures within bone tissue. These compounds work by

directly inhibiting the activity of the osteoclasts.

Bone density: The volume of calcium and minerals within the bone tissue, with the loss of these minerals resulting in osteoporosis.

Bone density test: Radiological technique for measuring the level of bone density at selected sites throughout the skeleton, or the total bone mass within the skeleton.

Bone formation-stimulating agent: An osteoporosis intervention intended to increase bone mass by increasing the bone remodeling rate and stimulating the activity of the osteoblasts.

Bone loss: The result of the body using calcium stored in bone without the ability to replace the minerals, decreasing the density of the bones.

Bone marrow: Found in the hollow cavities deep in the interior of bone, marrow is composed of blood vessels and a network of tissue fibers containing fat and the cells that produce blood.

Bone mass: The total amount of bone tissue in the skeleton.

Bone mineral content (BMC): A measurement of the total amount of mineral, including calcium, in bone.

Bone remodeling: The process by which bone is formed, broken down and formed again by the action of the osteoclasts and osteoblasts. Remodeling consists of three phases: resorption, formation and mineralization.

Bone resorption: The entire process in which the osteoclasts break down existing bone, releasing the calcium stored within to be reabsorbed into the bloodstream.

Bone turnover: The frequency with which bone is broken down and reformed by the remodeling process.

Calcitonin: A hormone produced by cells in the thyroid gland. Regulates the amount of calcium released from bone into the bloodstream, absorption of calcium in the digestive tract and its secretion by the kidneys. Used in osteoporosis intervention to repress osteoclast activity.

Calcitriol: An active form of vitamin D that increases absorption of calcium. Used as an osteoporosis intervention, calcitriol helps increase levels of calcium in the blood, which represses the production of parathyroid hormones.

Calcium: The mineral that makes up much of the physical composition of bone, and the most abundant mineral in the human body. Calcium phosphate crystals are embedded in the bone matrix through the *mineralization phase* of bone remodeling. Calcium provides strength and density to the bones, and the loss of calcium is what brings about the weakening of the skeleton that can lead to osteoporosis. Calcium is also a vital nutrient that performs several key functions throughout the body, such as proper clotting of the blood, normal functioning of muscles and nerves, and maintaining the heartbeat. About 99 percent of the body's calcium is stored in the skeleton.

Calcium excretion: The loss of calcium through the urine, feces and perspiration.

Calcium phosphate: A combination of calcium and phosphorus. Deposited from the bloodstream, calcium phosphate interweaves with the collagen matrix to mineralize new bone.

Carbohydrates: Foods that provide the primary source of energy for the body. Carbohydrates include sugars and starches. Up to 60 percent of the average American's diet consists of carbohydrates.

Cartilage: A fibrous, flexible tissue that forms the outer layer of bone at the joints. Cartilage plays an integral role in skeletal growth.

Cholesterol: A soft, waxy substance that is a member of the lipid family. It is one of the components of nerve linings, and is the substance from which the steroid hormones are formed, including estrogen, testosterone and vitamin D.

Collagen: A type of protein that forms many connective tissues of the human body; skin, cartilage and ligaments are made of collagen.

Cortical bone: The hard, dense outer shell of bone that makes up the bulk of the long bones found in the arms and legs. Also called compact bone.

Compression fracture: A break in a vertebra of the spine, in which the vertebra collapses. Also called a crush fracture.

Cyclical therapy: A form of drug therapy that incorporates an intermittent rest period in which the drug is not administered. In some cases another drug, vitamin or mineral (such as calcium) may be administered during the rest period. Many osteoporosis treatments use cyclical therapy.

Dowager's hump: A noticeable forward curvature of the spine caused by numerous vertebral fractures.

Dual energy X-ray absorptiometry (DEXA): An osteoporosis screening and diagnostic technique using X-rays filtered into two levels of energy, allowing fast and accurate measurement of bone density with minimal radiation exposure.

Early menopause: Onset of menopause before age 45. May occur naturally or as the result of surgical removal of the ovaries.

Electrolytes: Mineral compounds responsible for maintaining fluid balances and proper functioning of body cells. The primary electrolytes are sodium, potassium and chloride.

Endocrinology: The study of hormones and the organs and glands that produce them.

Epiphyseal growth plate: A thin disk of cartilage at the end of bone that is active during periods of longitudinal growth in childhood and adolescence. Adult height is reached when the growth plates stop functioning.

Estrogen: A family of hormones produced by the ovaries and testes. During adolescence, it stimulates growth of the long bones in women. Estrogen has a protective effect on bone mass, with the loss of estrogen at menopause resulting in a period of drastic bone loss.

Estrogen Replacement Therapy (ERT): Treatment that provides hormones lost when the ovaries halt production of estrogen, such as at menopause. ERT is one of the primary interventions for postmenopausal bone loss in women.

Etidronate: Also called etidronate disodium, a bisphosphonate drug approved by the FDA for the treatment of Paget's disease of the bone. The drug has also been used to treat osteoporosis.

Fat: The common term for the family of lipids. Some forms of fat are essential for life, performing vital functions throughout the body. Fat comprises a large part of cell membranes and nerve linings. Stored fat provides insulation against heat loss and protects bones and organs. Some bone-friendly hormones, such as estrogen, testosterone and vitamin D are manufactured from certain kinds of fats. Dietary fat provides taste and texture to many foods and is an important source of energy.

Fatty acids: Organic compounds made up primarily of carbon, hydrogen and oxygen molecules. Combinations of various fatty acids are the main component of fat.

Fiber: A form of carbohydrate found in a variety of substances, from apple pulp and citrus rind to wood chips and vegetable gums. Fiber is divided into two types: soluble fiber, which breaks down in water, and insoluble fiber, which does not.

Follicle-stimulating hormone (FSH): A hormone produced by the pituitary gland that stimulates the secretion of estrogen by the gonads. FSH is also a biochemical marker for estrogen deficiency, since production of this hormone increases as estrogen levels fall.

Fracture threshold: The level of bone density at which a person is in imminent danger of a spontaneous fracture.

Glucose: Blood sugar. Many tissues of the body, such as the brain, rely heavily on glucose for energy.

Hormones: Complex chemicals produced by glands and organs throughout the body. They are both catalysts and regulators of the most fundamental bodily functions, like heartbeat and digestion.

Hormone Replacement Therapy (HRT): A cyclical therapy that consists of about three weeks of estrogen followed by about two weeks of progestin. The therapy closely mimics the natural hormone cycle that occurs in menstruating women.

This facilitates the shedding of the uterine lining each month, believed by some experts to reduce the risk of uterine cancer associated with estrogen replacement therapy.

Hydrogenation: A process used by food manufacturers to make polyunsaturated fats hardy enough to withstand processing. The double carbon bonds of these fats are broken down and saturated with hydrogen. If not all of the double carbon bonds are broken, the product is *partially hydrogenated.*

Hypercalcemia: Excess calcium in the blood.

Intervention: In osteoporosis, treatment or therapy undertaken to reduce the rate of bone loss.

Lactose intolerance: An inability to digest the sugar in milk. People who lack an enzyme called **lactase** have difficulty breaking down lactose, and experience gastric disturbances like bloating, gas, cramps and diarrhea.

Ligaments: Bands of tissue that hold the joints of the bones together.

Lipoproteins: A combination of lipids and proteins that binds with cholesterol and carries it through the bloodstream. There are two types of lipoproteins: High density lipoproteins, or HDLs, help remove cholesterol from body tissues; low density lipoproteins, or LDLs, carry cholesterol that is more apt to adhere to the walls of arteries, increasing the risk of heart disease.

Menopause: The period in a woman's life when the ovaries have slowed production of estrogen and other female hormones. It begins when a woman has not experienced a menstrual flow for 12 consecutive months. The average American woman reaches menopause at around age 51.

Microfractures: Minuscule fissures in bone, sometimes called microcracks.

Mineralization: The phase of the bone remodeling process when calcium and phosphorus from the bloodstream interweave with the collagen matrix.

Minerals: Inorganic substances, over a dozen of which are known to be essential to life and health, with nearly twice that many forming the total mineral composition of the body. Minerals are generally needed in larger quantities than vitamins, and must come from dietary sources or supplements. Some of the vital minerals for which an RDA has been established are iron, magnesium, zinc, iodine, phosphorus and calcium.

Osteoblasts: The bone formation cells, which deposit a collagen matrix into the cavities in bone created by osteoclasts.

Osteoclasts: The cells that break down existing bone.

Osteitis fibrosa: A bone disease caused by an overactive parathyroid gland, which results in severe loss of bone mass.

Osteomalacia: See **Rickets**.

Osteoporosis: A condition that exists when loss of bone over time has caused the drastic weakening of the skeleton, and the bone density level has fallen below the fracture threshold.

Osteopenia: A condition characterized by loss of bone mass that has not yet reached the fracture threshold. Osteopenia is the precursor to osteoporosis.

Parathyroid hormone: A hormone that monitors the level of calcium in the blood. It is produced by the four tiny parathyroid glands near the thyroid in the neck. When there are insufficient levels of calcium in the bloodstream the parathyroid hormone stimulates the osteoclasts. This hormone helps convert vitamin D to an active form that increases dietary calcium absorption, and helps the kidneys metabolize calcium. Parathyroid hormone is under study as an intervention for bone loss.

Peak bone mass: The point in life at which bones are as dense and strong as they ever will be. This normally occurs between the ages of 15 and 20 to 25 in trabecular bone, and 25 to 35 in cortical bone.

Perimenopause: The period in which the ovaries are slowing their production of estrogen, with estrogen loss sometimes made evident by irregular periods and other symptoms associated with menopause. Perimenopause can last for several years, ending when a woman has her last menstrual period.

Periosteum: The thin, tough, protective membrane of fibrous tissue that encases bone and forms its outermost layer.

Physiatrist: A doctor who specializes in the diagnosis and treatment of muscle and skeletal disorders or diseases. Unlike orthopedic surgeons, physiatrists do not perform surgery. Physiatrists are heavily involved in rehabilitation therapies.

Physical therapist: While not a medical doctor, this specialist is generally licensed by the state and works closely with orthopedic surgeons and other medical professionals to design and implement a program for returning an injured or disabled patient to maximum physical capability.

Premature menopause: A condition in which the ovaries stop working, just as in normal menopause, except that the woman is much younger than the age when menopause is normally anticipated. (See **Early menopause**)

Progesterone: One of the key female sex hormones. It plays an important role in menstrual function and also protects bone mass.

Progestin: The synthetic form of progesterone used in hormone replacement therapy.

Protein: The substance that makes up much of the human body, and is used to grow, repair and maintain healthy tissue. Protein is made up of amino acids.

Resistance exercise: Exercise that utilizes an apparatus to make the muscles work harder to accomplish a task or motion.

Rickets: A condition in children characterized by the softening of the bones, resulting in deformities such as bow legs. In adults this condition is called osteomalacia, and is a breakdown in the mineralization process that hardens bone.

Salmon calcitonin: The form of calcitonin used in treating osteoporosis, manufactured to resemble the amino acid structure of calcitonin found in the salmon. Salmon calcitonin is about 50 times more potent in slowing bone resorption than that produced by the human thyroid.

Sex hormones: Hormones produced by the ovaries in females and the testes in males. The two primary female sex hormones, estrogen and progesterone, act as bone protectors and prevent adrenal hormones from destroying bone. Sex hormones like estrogen, progesterone and, in males, androgens stimulate rapid growth in adolescence.

Sodium fluoride: A compound commonly added to drinking water and toothpaste to strengthen teeth. It has emerged as a potent bone formation-stimulating agent in the treatment of osteoporosis. Initial positive results have been tempered by the discovery that new bone formed as a result of sodium fluoride therapy is inferior to normal bone.

Steroids: Hormones produced by various glands on an "as needed" basis from cholesterol in the bloodstream. Estrogen, testosterone and the adrenal hormones are steroids, as is vitamin D.

Surgical menopause: A physical condition with the attributes of natural menopause; due to the loss of hormones as a result of surgical removal of the ovaries, medically known as an *oophorectomy*. Usually done along with a *hysterectomy*, which is the removal of the uterus and possibly the cervix.

Tendons: Strong cord-like fibrous tissues that attach the muscles to bones.

Thiazide diuretics: Drugs used in the treatment of high blood pressure and other circulatory problems. Used as an intervention for bone loss after researchers discovered that thiazide increases the amount of calcium in the bloodstream.

Trabecular bone: Also called cancellous bone; the soft, spongy, porous bone tissue that makes up a large part of the vertebrae and ribs. Trabecular bone is the more metabolically active form of bone tissue.

Vitamin D: Both a steroid hormone and a vitamin, it is one of the key components in forming healthy bone. It helps increase intestinal absorption of dietary calcium and aids the reabsorption of calcium in the kidneys.

Vitamins: Organic substances the body requires in tiny amounts for healthy functioning. These micronutrients cannot be manufactured by the body and thus must be supplied in the diet.

Select Bibliography

The references listed here are not a complete record of all works used in researching this book. Rather, they are given as sources that may be of particular interest to those who wish to pursue further specific issues pertaining to osteoporosis.

Books

"Bones." *Encyclopaedia Britannica.* 15th ed. Chicago: Encyclopaedia Britannica Inc., 1991.

Cooper, K.H. *Preventing Osteoporosis.* New York: Bantam, 1989.

Henig, R.M. *How A Woman Ages.* New York: Ballantine Books/Random House, 1985.

Miller, B.F. and Brackman, C.K. *Encyclopedia & Dictionary of Medicine and Nursing.* Philadelphia: W.B. Saunders Company, 1972.

Notelovitz, Morris. *Stand Tall: Every Woman's Guide To Preventing Osteoporosis.* New York: Bantam, 1985.

Government Documents

U.S. Congress. House Subcommittee On Human Services of the Select Committee On Aging. *International Perspectives On Osteoporosis.* May 1989. 101st Cong., 1st sess., 1989. H.Doc. 101-713.

U.S. Department of Agriculture and U.S. Department of Health and Human Services. *Nutrition and Your Health: Dietary Guidelines for Americans.* Washington, D.C.: GPO, 1985.

U.S. Department of Health and Human Services. *Osteoporosis Research, Education and Health Promotion.* Washington, D.C.: GPO, 1990.

Journal Articles

Chestnut, C.H. III. "Osteoporosis and Its Treatment." *New England Journal of Medicine* 326(February 1992): 406-409.

Goodman, C.E. "Osteoporosis: Protective Measures of Nutrition and Exercise." *Geriatrics* 40(1985): 59-70.

Johnston, C.C. Jr., Longscope, C. "Premenopausal Bone Loss — A Risk Factor for Osteoporosis." *New England Journal of Medicine* 323(November 1990): 1271-1274.

Kelsey, J., Hoffman, S. "Risk Factors for Hip Fracture." *New England Journal of Medicine* 316(1987): 404.

Lindsay, R. "Fluoride and Bone — Quantity vs Quality." *New England Journal of Medicine* 322(March 1990): 845-847.

Meredith, C.N. "Dietary Measures to Decrease Disability in Elderly Women." *Nutrition & The M.D.* 19(January 1993): 1-4.

Nordin, B.E.C. "The Definition and Diagnosis of Osteoporosis." *California Tissue International* 40(1987): 57.

Prince, R.L., Smith, M., Dick, I.M., et al. "Prevention of Postmenopausal Osteoporosis: A Comparative Study of Exercise, Calcium Supplementation and Hormone Replacement Therapy." *New England Journal of Medicine* 325(1991): 1189-1195.

Riggs, B.L. "A New Option for Treating Osteoporosis." *New England Journal of Medicine* 323(July 1990): 124-126.

Riggs, B.L., Hodgson, S.F., O'Fallon, W.M., et al. "Effect of Fluoride Treatment on the Fracture Rate in Postmenopausal Women with Osteoporosis." *New England Journal of Medicine* 322(1990): 802-809.

Riggs, B.L., Melton, L.J. "Involutional Osteoporosis." *New England Journal of Medicine* 314(1986): 1676-1685.

Smith, E.L. "How Exercise Helps Prevent Osteoporosis." *Contemporary OB/GYN* 25(1985): 51-60.

Urrows, S.T., Freston, M.S. "Profiles in Osteoporosis." *American Journal of Nursing,* 91(December 1991): 32-40.

U.S. Department of Agriculture and U.S. Department of Health and Human Services. *Nutrition and Your Health: Dietary Guidelines for Americans.* Washington, D.C.: GPO, 1985.

Watts, N.B., Harris, S.T., et al. "Intermittent Cyclical Etidronate Treatment of Postmenopausal Osteoporosis." *New England Journal of Medicine* 323(July 1990): 73-80.

Magazine Articles

Altman, L.K. "New Therapy Shown to Fight Bone Loss in Elderly." *New York Times,* 12 July 1990, A1.

Amato, I. "Growth-hormone Levels Plummet in Space." *Science News,* 1 September 1990, 134.

"Another Challenge to Coffee's Safety." *Science News,* 20 October 1990, 253.

Attie, M. "Bisphosphonate Therapy for Osteoporosis." *Hospital Practice,* 30 March 1991, 87-90.

"Belief in Boron: An Element of Strength." *Science News,* 1 April 1989, 204.

Brady, D. "Brittle Bones." *Maclean's,* 23 July 1990, 38.

Devereaux, K. "Calcium Tablets: Bone Up On the Basics." *Women's Sports & Fitness*, May 1989, 22.

Fackelmann, K.A. "Bone Loss Tied to Autoimmune Reaction." *Science News*, 7 March 1992, 159.

Findlay, S., Linnon, N., et al. "Almanac." *U.S. News & World Report*, 18 June 1990, 76.

Fletcher, A. "Healthy Bones Year after Year from the National Osteoporosis Foundation." *Prevention*, November 1990, 47.

"For Older Women, Calcium Counts." *Newsweek*, 8 October 1990, 77.

Gutfeld, G. "Kids May Bank Bone." *Prevention*, August 1990, 10-12.

Gutfeld, G. "Less Salt, More Bone?" *Prevention*, October 1991, 10.

Hunter, B.T. "Food Health Claims: Fact vs. Fiction." *Consumers' Research Magazine*, May 1991, 10-15.

McVeigh, G. "On the Trail of Nutrition's White Knight." *Prevention*, February 1990, 60-68.

"New Hope for Old Bones." *Newsweek*, 14 May 1990, 55.

Podolsky, K., MacMillan, J. "Eat Your Beans." *U.S. News & World Report*, 20 May 1991, 70-71.

Raloff, J. "Bone Savers: Rating Lifestyle and Drugs." *Science News*, 26 October 1991, 262-263.

"Score Three for Longevity." *U.S. News & World Report*, 31 December 1990, 64.

Stolzenburg, W. "Hard Evidence for Bone-building Therapy." *Science News*, 14 July 1990, 22.

"Strengthening Bones Without Hormones." *Science News*, 26 May 1990, 334.

"The Heart of the Matter." *U.S. News & World Report*, 5 August 1991, 10.

Newsletter Articles

"Fracture study with alendronate largest to date." *SCRIP World Pharmaceutical News* No. 1775, PJB Publications, Ltd., 1 December 1992, 24.

"Italian tamoxifen prophylaxis trial." *SCRIP World Pharmaceutical News* No. 1773, PJB Publications, Ltd., 24 November 1992, 26.

"Lilly's novel approach to osteoporosis." and "New data on Merck's alendronate." *SCRIP World Pharmaceutical News* No. 1812/13, PJB Publications, Ltd., 16/20 April 1993, 30-31.

"Oestrogen gel nearing UK market?" *SCRIP World Pharmaceutical News* No. 1814, PJB Publications, Ltd., 23 April 1993, 31.

"Oestrogen plus fluoride for osteoporosis?" *SCRIP World Pharmaceutical News* No. 1814, PJB Publications, Ltd., 23 April 1993, 31.

"Osteoporosis consensus statement emphasises prevention." *SCRIP World Pharmaceutical News* No. 1810/11, PJB Publications, Ltd., 9/13 April 1993, 34.

Newspaper Articles

Hellmich, N. "Pumping Iron May Be Key To Enjoying the Golden Years." *USA Today*, 25 February 1993, 5D.

Hellmich, N. "Ways To Make Exercising A Family Affair." *USA Today*, 24 March 1993, 5D.

Organization Pamphlets

American College of Sports Medicine. *What Is An Exercise Physiologist?* Indianapolis: American College of Sports Medicine.

Every Woman's Guide to Health and Nutrition. Rosemont: National Dairy Council, 1988.

For Mature Eaters Only: Guidelines for Good Nutrition. Rosemont: National Dairy Council, 1989.

Johnston, C.C., Christiansen, C., Lindsay, R., and Marcus, R. *Osteoporosis Update: Highlights from the 1990 International Council on Menopause Therapy.* Medical Education Programs, Ltd., 1991.

National Dairy Board. *Dairy: The Backbone of Every Woman's Diet.* Rosemont: National Dairy Board, 1986.

National Dairy Council. *Calcium: You Never Outgrow Your Need For It.* Rosemont: National Dairy Council, 1984.

National Osteoporosis Foundation. *Boning Up On Osteoporosis: A Guide To Prevention and Treatment.* Washington, D.C.: National Osteoporosis Foundation, 1991.

National Osteoporosis Foundation. *Can It Happen To You?* Washington, D.C.: National Osteoporosis Foundation, 1991.

National Osteoporosis Foundation. *Osteoporosis: A Woman's Guide.* Washington, D.C.: National Osteoporosis Foundation, 1988.

Wyeth-Ayerst Laboratories. *What You Should Know About Estrogen Deficiency and Osteoporosis.* Philadelphia: Wyeth-Ayerst Laboratories, 1991.

Index

A

Absorptiometry, 54, 61-62,
    See also Bone density
    measurement
Absorption, 25, 176
Active vitamin D, 99-100
Adolescence, 19-20, 167
Adrenal glands, 68
Adrenal hormones, 17
Adrenaline, 68
Aerobic exercise, 110, 111-
    112, 135-137
Aging, 10-11, 21-22, 25, 27-
    28, 85, 169, *See also* Elderly
Alcohol use, 34, 209-210
Alendronate, 98-99
Almond Coffee Cake, 193
Amenorrhea, 28, 73, 124, 202
American Association of
    Retired Persons (AARP),
    217
American Medical
    Association, 89
Amino acids, 155
Anabolic metabolism, 68
Anabolic steroids, 101
Androgens, 68-69, 71, 101
Androsterone, 69
Anorexia nervosa, 28, 202
Antacids, 11, 176
Anti-estrogens, 103, 105-106
Anti-resorptive agents, 92,
    See also Drug therapy
Appetizer recipes, 179-180
Arthritis, 34, 207
Athletics, 114-115,
    See also Exercise

B

Back pain, 50
Balance problems, 208-209
Bean Soup, 183-184
Berry Delight, 182
Beverage recipes, 181-182, 203
Bioavailable calcium, 175
Biochemical markers, 62
Bisphosphonates, 96-99
Blood cell production, 15
Blood clotting, 81, 82
Blood pressure, 81
Blood tests, 50-51, 62-64
Blue Cross and Blue Shield,
    45

Body size, 31
Bone density, 3, 15, 17-25,
    See also Bone loss; Bone
    mass
Bone density measurement,
    10, 42-43
    diagnostic tests, 42, 49-51
    methods, 54-56, 60-63
    National Osteoporosis
        Foundation guidelines, 47
    patient experiences, 58-60
    peak bone mass determina-
        tions, 19
    screening tests, 42-49
    See also Testing
Bone-destroying cells,
    See Osteoclasts
Bone diseases, 28
Bone formation, 18-21, 71,
    See also Bone remodeling
Bone formation-stimulating
    agents, 92-93, 102, 103-106
Bone-forming cells,
    See Osteoblasts
Bone loss, 3, 43
    age and, 21-22, 25, 27
    estrogen replacement and,
        79-80
    exercise and, 36, 108-110
    inactivity and, 10, 25, 108,
        111
    menopause effects, 9-10,
        22-25, 27, 31
    salt and, 163
Bone marrow, 15
Bone mass, 15, 176
    estrogen deficiency and, 73
    peak, 19-20, 195
    therapeutic increase, 88, 95
Bone mineral content (BMC),
    43-44, 54, 57, 59
Bone remodeling, 13, 16-18,
    92, *See also* Mineralization
Bone resorption, 16, 87, 92,
    104, 166
Bone scan, 54
Bone turnover, 18, 21, 63
Bowel disorders, 32
Bread Rolls, 180
Breast cancer, 76, 80, 105-106
Breast-feeding, 37, 81, 167
Broccoli Stir-fry, 192
Broccoli-stuffed Pasta, 188

Bulimia, 28
Burrito recipe, 204
Butler, Sheri, 120, 122, 200

C

Caesar Salad, 186-187
Caffeine, 35, 175
Calcitonin, 17, 68, 86, 94-96
Calcitriol, 99-100
Calcium, 9-11, 25, 37-38, 89,
    93-94
    absorption of, 25, 176
    bone remodeling process,
        16-17
    caffeine and, 35
    child and adolescent diets,
        197-199
    excretion of, 93, 100, 174-
        175
    food groups, 169-174
    recommended intake, 11,
        167-169, 199
    side effects, 94
    skeletal storage, 14, 166-167
    smoking and, 36
    supplements, 7, 11, 37, 94,
        175-178
Calcium carbonate, 177, 178
Calcium citrate, 178
Calcium gluconate, 178
Calcium lactate, 178
Calcium phosphate, in bone,
    13-14, 37, 43, 93
Calcium phosphate
    supplement, 177
Calcium-rich recipes,
    179-194
    appetizers, 179-180
    beverages, 181-182, 203
    desserts, 193-194, 204-205
    entrees, 188-190
    for children, 203-206
    salads, 185-187
    soups, 183-185
    vegetables, 191-192
Calcium robbers, 174-175
Calisthenics, 112, 113, 149-
    152
Calorie, 154
Cancer, 41, 75, 76, 80
Carbohydrates, 160-161
Carbonated beverages, 39,
    175

Cardiovascular disease, 76
Cardiovascular system, 111
Cartilage, 13-14
Catabolic metabolism, 68
CAT scan, 54, 59, 61
Cellulose, 164
Cheese, 11, 172-183, 180, 191-192
Cheesecake, 193-194
Chelated calcium, 178
Chicken Enchiladas, 188-189
Children, 9, 18-19, 29, 195-196
  exercise program for, 121, 200-201
  nutrition for, 196-200, 203-206
Chili recipe, 184-185
Cholesterol, 161-162, 197
Cigarette smoking, 11, 35-36
Climacteric symptoms, 22
Clinical trials, 7, 90, 99
Clodronate, 98
Clotting problems, 81, 82
Cocoa, 203
Coffee Cake, 193
Collagen, 16
Colorful Vegetable Bake, 191
Complete protein, 156
Complex carbohydrates, 160-161
Conjugated equine estrogen, 77
Controllable risk factors, 34-39
Cool-down exercise, 113, 125
Corpus luteum, 70
Cortical bone, 14, 19, 95, 102, 104
Corticosteroids, 33-34, 99
Cortisone, 68
Costs, *See* Economic costs
Cottage Cheesecake, 193-194
Cream of Broccoli Soup, 183
Cross-training, 114, 143
Cyclical therapy, 95, 97

D

Densitometry, *See* Bone density measurement
Density, *See* Bone density
Depression, 72-73
Dessert recipes, 193-194, 204-205

Diagnostic tests, 42, 49-51, *See also* Bone density measurement
Diet, *See* Nutrition
Digestive disorders, 32
Diphosphonates, 96-99
Diseases, 28
Diuretics, 100
Doctor-patient partnership, 83-84, 88-89
Dolomite, 176
Dowager's hump, 5, 49
DPA, 61
Drug resistance, 95
Drug therapy, 87-89
  anabolic steroids, 101
  bisphosphonates, 96-99
  calcitonin, 68, 86, 94-96
  calcitriol, 99-100
  costs of, 95, 97
  experimental drugs, 92-93, 103-106
  FDA approval, 86, 90-91, 98
  fluoride, 101-103
  growth factors, 104-105
  mode of action, 91-93
  parathyroid hormone, 103-104
  raloxifene, 106
  side effects, 101
  tamoxifen, 105-106
  testosterone, 74, 101
  thiazide diuretics, 100
  See also specific drugs and hormones
Dual Photon Absorptiometry (DPA), 61
Dual X-Ray Absorptiometry (DEXA), 62

E

Ear disorders, 209
Early menopause, 31, 35-36, 73-74
Eating disorders, 28, 202
Economic costs:
  bone density tests, 45, 47, 56-58, 61
  drug therapies, 95, 97
  insurance coverage, 45, 58, 61
Education, 8-9
Elderly, 10-11, 25
  calcium needs, 169
  exercise programs, 123
  See also Aging

Electrolytes, 165-166
Emotional problems, 72-73
Emotional stress, 36-37, 73, 110
Enchiladas, 188-189
Endocrinologists, 53
Endocrinology, 65-69
Endometrium, 70
Entree recipes, 188-190
Environmental hazards, 211-214
Epinephrine, 68
Epiphyseal growth plates, 14
ERT, *See* Estrogen replacement therapy
Essential amino acids, 155
Estradiol, 78
Estrogen, 66, 69-71
  deficiency, 24, 73-74
  excess exercise and, 28, 73, 124, 202
  fat and, 23, 31, 202
  menopause and, 22-25, 31, 71
  receptors, 105
  smoking and, 35-36
Estrogen analogues, 103, 105-106
Estrogen patches, 77-78
Estrogen replacement therapy (ERT), 24-25, 74-84
  alternative treatments, 89-106
  calcium intake recommendations, 168-169
  contraindications, 81-82
  effectiveness of, 79-80
  FDA approval, 86
  formulations, 77-78
  progestin cotherapy, 75
  risks, 75, 76, 80-81
  side effects, 75, 82
Etidronate, 96-98
Excretion, calcium, 93, 100, 174-175
Exercise, 9, 10, 28, 36, 108-112
  adult programs, 122-123
  calisthenics, 113, 149-152
  for children, 121, 200-201
  health professionals, 116-117
  injury prevention benefits, 209
  intensity, 110, 111, 135
  low bone density and, 117

menstrual effects, 28, 73, 124, 202
motivation level for, 115-116
resistance, 112-113, 141-149
stretching, 113, 125-127
target heart rate, 118-119
walking, 115-116, 129-132
warning signs, 120
weight-bearing, 112, 128-140
Exercise physiologist, 117
Experimental drugs, 92-93, 103-106

F
Falls, 10, 12, 25, 207-214
Family history, 31
Family practice physicians, 53
Fat, 23, 31, 157-159, 202
Fatty acids, 157-158
FDA approval, 86, 90-91, 98
Fetal growth, 18-19
FIT formula, 129
Fleisch, Herbert, 96
Flexion exercises, 117
Floor exercises, 149
Fluoride, 101-103
Follicle-stimulating hormone (FSH), 67, 73
Follow-up, 48, 55, 63
Food and Drug Administration (FDA), 86, 90-91, 98
Food groups, 169-174
Foot care, 131, 210
Forearm bone, 55, 59, 60
Fracture(s), 3-6, *See also* Hip fractures; Vertebral fractures
estrogen replacement and, 79
prediction of, 47
Fracture Intervention Trial (FIT), 99
Fracture threshold, 3, 11, 29, 43
Frozen Orange Yogurt, 205-206
Frozen Peach Pops, 206
Fruits, 172
Fruit salad, 185-186
FSH, 67, 73

G
Gallbladder disease, 80
Garden Burrito, 204
Gender, as osteoporosis risk factor, 30
Geriatricians, 53
Glucocorticoids, 68

Glucose, 160
Gonads, 69
Government programs, 215-216
Growth factors, 104-105
Growth hormone, 17
Gynecologists, 53

H
Health insurance, 45-46, 58, 61
Heart rate, 118-119
Hearty Bean Soup, 183-184
Heel bone, 55, 59, 60
Height, 5, 49
High-density lipoproteins (HDL), 162, 163
Hip, bone density measurement, 59
Hip fractures, 3, 5-6, 29, 30, 51, 79
Home safety, 211-214
Hormone(s), 17-18, 65-69, 91, *See also* Estrogen; *other specific hormones*
Hormone replacement therapy, 7, 75, *See also* Estrogen replacement therapy
Hospitals, 218
Hot cocoa, 203
Hot flashes, 72
Human calcitonin, 95
Hydrogenation, 159
Hyperparathyroidism, 47
Hypertension, 81
Hypothalamus, 67
Hysterectomy, 23

I
Impact, 114, 136
Inactivity, 10, 25, 108, 111
Individualized treatment, 88
Information resources, 215-218
Injury prevention, 10, 12, 207-214, 217
Insoluble fiber, 164
Insulin, 160
Insurance coverage, 45, 58, 61
Intensity, 110, 111, 135
Internists, 53
Intervention, 87, *see also* Treatment
Intestinal disorders, 32
Iron supplement, 177
Isotopes, 54, 61

JKL
Jogging, 113, 128
Johnston, C. Conrad, Jr., 56, 79, 89, 197
Jumping rope, 134-135
Kidneys, 32, 67, 100
Lactase, 174
Lactose intolerance, 38, 174
Landers, Ann, 1-2
Lang, Robert, 48, 62, 88
Laxatives, 177
Lifestyle risk factors, 25-26, 34-39
Lifting, 210, 212
Ligaments, 13
Lighting, 211
Lipids, 157
Lipoproteins, 161-162
Lite and Lean Nachos, 179
Liver disease, 32, 80, 82
Longitudinal bone growth, 14
Long-term care, 6
Low-density lipoproteins (LDL), 162, 163
Lower back pain, 50
Lupus, 82

M
Male menopause, 74
Male osteoporosis patients, 6, 34, 89
Manganese, 94
Marrow, 15
Marvelous Meatless Chili, 184-185
Meat, 11, 172
Meatloaf, 204
Medicare coverage, 45-46, 58, 60, 61
Medication, 29, 33-34, *See also* Drug therapy
calcium supplement interactions, 176
falling, dangers from, 207, 208-209
Medulla, 68
Menopause, 9-10, 22-25, 27, 31, 71-73
calcium intake recommendations, 168-169
demographic effects, 85
male, 74
premature, 31, 35-36, 73-74
smoking and, 35-36
surgical, 23, 31

Menstruation:
  estrogen levels and, 70
  excessive exercise and, 28, 73, 124, 202-203
  See also Menopause
Metabolism, 68
Michigan Meatloaf, 204
Migraine, 82
Milk products, 38, 172-174, 205-206
Mineralization, 17, 93, 97, 167
  bone disease and, 28
  fluoride effects, 102
  loss of, 22
Minerals, 164-166
Mocha Instant Breakfast, 182
Mood swings, 72
Motivation, 115-116
Mozzarella Snacks, 180
Muscles, 13

N
Nachos, 177
Nasal spray, 95-96
National Institutes of Health (NIH), 85-86, 106, 216
National Osteoporosis Foundation, 4, 8, 45, 47, 216
Nursing home care, 6
Nutrition, 9-11, 29, 37-39, 153-155
  calcium-rich recipes, 179-194
  calcium robbers, 174-175
  carbohydrates, 160-161
  for children, 9, 196-200, 203-206
  cholesterol, 161-162
  fat, 157-159
  food groups, 169-174
  injury prevention and, 210
  protein, 155-157
  sodium, 163-163
  vitamins and minerals, 164-166
  See also Calcium; *specific foods and nutrients*

O
Old-Fashioned Hot Cocoa, 203
Oophorectomy, 23
Oriental Omelet, 189-190
Orthopedic surgeons, 53
Os calcis, 55, 59, 60
Osteitis fibrosa, 28

Osteoblasts, 16, 92, 166
  calcitriol effects, 100
  estrogen and, 71
  fluoride effects, 102
  growth factors and, 104
Osteoclasts, 16, 87, 92
  bisphosphonate effects, 96
  blood-calcium levels and, 166
  estrogen and, 23
  hormone effects on, 17, 104
Osteomalacia, 28
Osteopenia, 29, 43
Osteoporosis, 2-4, 6
  male sufferers, 6, 34, 89
  reversibility of, 88
  types of, 3, 24
  warning signs, 4, 50
Osteoporosis risk, *See* Risk factors
Osteoporosis treatment, *See* Treatment
Ovaries, 23, 69
Ovulation, 70
Oxalates, 175
Oxytocin, 67

P
Pain, 50, 94
Pamidronate, 98
Pap smear, 41
Parathyroid disease, 32, 47
Parathyroid gland, 28, 68, 103-104
Parathyroid hormone (PTH), 17, 68, 71, 104
Parkinson's disease, 208
Partially hydrogenated oils, 159
Patient bill of rights, 89
Peak bone mass, 19-20, 195
Perimenopause, 9-10, 71
Periosteum, 13
Phosphorus, 17, 38-39
Physiatrist, 117
Physical therapist, 117
Phytates, 175
Pineapple Chicken, 190
Pituitary gland, 67
Polyunsaturated fats, 159, 162
Pregnancy, 37, 69, 81, 167
Premature menopause, 31, 35-36, 73-74
Prevention, 8-12
  of falls and injuries, 207-214
  insurance coverage for, 45-46, 58

  See also Exercise; Nutrition; Testing
Primary hyperparathyroidism, 47
Primary osteoporosis, 3, 24
Progesterone, 22, 23, 31, 69, 70, 75
Progestin, 75
Protein, 155-157, 175
Puberty, 70
Public health policy, 85-86
Pulse point, 118

QR
QCT, 54, 59, 61
Quantitative Computed Tomography (QCT), 54, 59, 61
Race, 31
Radial artery, 118-119
Radiation dose, 61
Radioactive isotopes, 54
Radiology, 54
Radius bone, 55, 59, 60
Raloxifene, 106
Receptors, 66, 105
Recipes, *See* Calcium-rich recipes
Recommended Daily Allowances, 94, 154
Recommended Dietary Allowances, 154
Red marrow, 15
Refreshing Fruit Salad, 185-186
Remodeling, *See* Bone remodeling
Renal hypercalciuria, 100
Repetitions, 142
Residronate, 98
Resistance exercise, 112-113, 141-149
Resorption, 16, *See also* Bone resorption
Resources, 52-53, 215-218
Rheumatologists, 53
Rickets, 28
Riggs, B. Lawrence, 8, 12, 58, 102-103, 105, 108, 196
Risk factors, 27-30
  assessment quiz, 39-40
  controllable, 34-38
  testing guidelines, 47
  unavoidable, 30-34
Running, 113, 128

S

Safety, 207-214
Salad recipes, 185-187
Salmon calcitonin, 86, 95
Salmon Macaroni Salad, 187
Salt, 39, 162-163, 175
Saturated fats, 157-158, 162
Screening tests, 42-49, *See also* Bone density measurement
Seasoned Mozzarella Snacks, 180
Secondary osteoporosis, 3, 24
Secondary sex characteristics, 70
Sedentary lifestyle, 10, 25, 108, 111
Self-help organizations, 218
Semicircular canals, 209
Sex hormones, 17-18, 67-69, *See also specific hormones*
Sexual development, 70
Sexual intercourse, 72
Side effects, 82, 101
Single Photon Absorptiometry (SPA), 60
Single-site measurement, 55
Skeletal fitness, 111-115, *See also* Exercise
Skeletal system, 13-17, *See also specific bone entries*
Skin problems, 72
Smoking, 11, 35-36
Social Security Administration, 217
Socioeconomic impacts, 6
Sodium, 162-163
Sodium fluoride, 101-103
Soluble fiber, 163-164
Somatotropin, 67
Soup recipes, 183-185
Spaghetti Squash Mozzarella, 191-192
Special Baked Apple, 194
Specialists, 52-53, 116-117
Spine, 15, 59
    vertebral fractures, 3-5, 49, 51, 79, 97, 99
Sports, 114-115
Stair climbing, 133-134
Starches, 160
Stationary cycling, 128, 137-140
Steroids, 67, 101
Stomach disorders, 32
Strength training, 141
Stress, 36-37, 73, 110

Stretching, 113, 125-127
Stuffed Bread Rolls, 180
Sugars, 160, 161
Sunlight exposure, 11, 38
Support groups, 218
Surgical menopause, 23, 31
Swimming, 114

T

Tamoxifen, 105-106
Target heart rate, 118-120
Teenagers, *See* Adolescence
Tendons, 13
Testes, 69
Testing:
    blood and urine, 50-51, 62-64
    bone turnover, 63
    costs for, 45, 47, 56-58
    diagnostic, 42, 49-51
    estrogen deficiency, 73
    follow-up, 48, 55, 63
    insurance coverage for, 45-46, 58, 61
    screening, 42-49
    single-site measurement, 55
    See also Bone density measurement
Testosterone, 36, 69, 74, 101
Thiazide diuretics, 100
Thromboembolic disease, 81
Thyroid disease, 32
Thyroid gland, 68
Thyroid hormones, 17, 33
Tiludronate, 98
Tobacco smoking, 11, 35-36
Trabecular bone, 14
    calcitonin therapy, 95
    density measurement, 55
    fluoride effects, 101-102
    parathyroid hormone effects, 104
    peak bone mass, 195
Trace elements, 166
Transdermal patches, 78
Treatment, 87-89
    costs of, 95, 97
    resources and specialists, 52-53
Women's Health Initiative, 7
    See also Calcium; Drug therapy; Estrogen replacement therapy
Tropical oils, 158
Tropical Teaser, 181
Turkey Taco Casserole, 205

Type I osteoporosis, 3, 24
Type II osteoporosis, 3, 24

UV

Unsaturated fatty acids, 157-158
Urinary excretion, 93, 100, 174
Urinary tract infections, 72
Urine testing, 50-51, 62-64
Uterine cancer, 41, 75, 80
Vaginal bleeding, 82
Vegetables, 171, 191-192
Vegetarian diets, 29, 38
Vertebrae, 15
Vertebral fractures, 3-5, 49, 51, 97, 99
Vision impairment, 207, 209
Vitamins, 164-165
Vitamin D, 38, 67, 165, 169
    absorption impairment, 25
    active form, 99-100
    postmenopause prevention program, 10
    smoking and, 36
    supplements, 7, 93
    osteoporosis prevention program, 11

WXY

Walking, 115-116, 129-132
Warm-up exercise, 113, 125
Warning signs, 4, 50, 120
Water pills, 100
Weight-bearing exercise, 112, 128-140
Weight machines, 142
Weight-supported exercise, 114
Weight training, *See* Resistance exercise
Women's health centers, 218
Women's Health Initiative, 6-7, 85-86, 106
Wrist fractures, 3-4, 79
X-rays, 50, 54, 62
Yellow marrow, 15
Yogurt, 172, 174, 205-206